Cleveland Cli
of Vascular S

Samir K. Shah • Daniel G. Clair
Editors

Cleveland Clinic Manual of Vascular Surgery

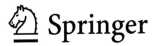 Springer

Editors
Samir K. Shah
Department of General Surgery
The Cleveland Clinic Foundation
Cleveland, OH, USA

Daniel G. Clair
Department of Vascular Surgery
The Cleveland Clinic Foundation
Cleveland, OH, USA

ISBN 978-1-4939-1630-6   ISBN 978-1-4939-1631-3 (eBook)
DOI 10.1007/978-1-4939-1631-3
Springer New York Heidelberg Dordrecht London

Library of Congress Control Number: 2014950408

Printed on acid-free paper

Springer is part of Springer Science+Business Media (www.springer.com)

Preface

Vascular surgery is a field of immense, sometimes overwhelming, breadth and depth. More than most disciplines, vascular surgery continues to grow rapidly, especially with the ongoing development of endovascular techniques. Fortunately, there are several authoritative textbooks that successfully catalog this knowledge but none does so concisely in a format convenient for the busy clinician caring for the vascular patient. The *Cleveland Clinic Manual of Vascular Surgery* is intended to fill this gap. The Cleveland Clinic has a rich tradition of treating cardiovascular disease, from F. Mason Sones' discovery of coronary angiography and Rene Favaloro's first coronary artery bypass graft to pioneering endovascular therapy for complex aortic disease. The knowledge gleaned from this long history has been distilled in the chapters that follow by the staff at the Cleveland Clinic. We have also incorporated vascular surgery fellowship graduates who currently hold staff positions across the country. It is our hope that we have balanced brevity with comprehensiveness in a way that principally helps vascular surgery fellows and residents but should be of value to anyone who may be involved in the care of vascular disease, including those in the fields of cardiology, interventional radiology, general surgery, and vascular medicine.

Cleveland, OH, USA

Samir K. Shah
Daniel G. Clair

Contents

Part III   Miscellaneous

Contributors

Julie E. Adams, M.D. Department of Surgery, Fletcher Allen Health Care, Burlington, VT, USA

Javier A. Alvarez-Tostado, M.D. Department of Vascular Surgery, Cleveland Clinic, Garfield, Heights, OH, USA

Daniel G. Clair, M.D. Department of Vascular Surgery, The Cleveland Clinic Foundation, Cleveland, OH, USA

Masato Fujiki, M.D., Ph.D. Department of General Surgery, Transplantation Center, Cleveland Clinic, Cleveland, OH, USA

Ramyar Gilani, M.D. Division of Vascular Surgery, Baylor College of Medicine, Houston, TX, USA

Michael E. DeBakey Department of Surgery, Baylor College of Medicine, Houston, TX, USA

Koji Hashimoto, M.D., Ph.D. Department of General Surgery, Transplantation Center, Cleveland Clinic, Cleveland, OH, USA

Jeanwan Kang, M.D. Department of Vascular Surgery, Cleveland Clinic, Cleveland, OH, USA

Lee Kirksey, M.D. Department of Vascular Surgery, Cleveland Clinic, Cleveland, OH, USA

Carol A. Langford, M.D., M.H.S. Department of Rheumatic and Immunologic Diseases, Center for Vasculitis Care and Research, Cleveland Clinic, Cleveland, OH, USA

Sean P. Lyden Department of Vascular Surgery, Cleveland Clinic, Cleveland, OH, USA

Charles Miller, M.D. Department of General Surgery, Transplantation Center, Cleveland Clinic, Cleveland, OH, USA

Samir K. Shah, M.D. Department of General Surgery, The Cleveland Clinic Foundation, Cleveland, OH, USA

Christopher J. Smolock, M.D. Department of Vascular Surgery, Cleveland Clinic, Cleveland, OH, USA

Lina M. Vargas, M.D. Department of Thoracic and Cardiovascular Surgery, Heart and Vascular Institute, Cleveland Clinic, Cleveland, OH, USA

Part I
Arterial Aneurysms

Chapter 1
Abdominal Aortic Aneurysm

Christopher J. Smolock and Sean P. Lyden

Introduction

Abdominal aortic aneurysm (AAA) is defined as focal dilation of the juxtarenal or infrarenal aorta having a 50 % increase in diameter compared to the expected normal diameter aorta in question. Normal size range of the abdominal aorta by cadaveric studies, angiography, computed tomography (CT), and duplex studies is 10–24 mm. Etiology is degenerative/atherosclerotic, inflammatory, degeneration after dissection, trauma, infection, or congenital. Degenerative infrarenal aortic aneurysms are the most common type of aneurysm of the aorta.

Demographics and Clinical Presentation

The true incidence of ruptured abdominal aortic aneurysms is difficult to determine but varies anywhere between 2 and 15 admissions per 100,000 patients depending on the population. The prevalence estimate for asymptomatic AAA in patients >50 years old is 3–10 %.

C.J. Smolock, M.D. (✉) • S.P. Lyden
Department of Vascular Surgery, Cleveland Clinic,
9500 Euclid Avenue, H32, Cleveland, OH 44195, USA
e-mail: smolocc@ccf.org; smolock1@gmail.com

S.K. Shah and D.G. Clair (eds.), *Cleveland Clinic Manual of Vascular Surgery*, DOI 10.1007/978-1-4939-1631-3_1,
© Springer Science+Business Media New York 2014

In addition to presenting as acute rupture, AAAs often present as incidental findings on a variety of imaging studies performed for other indications. Atheroembolism and, less commonly, thrombosis occur in <5 % of patients with AAA and such an etiology must be considered as a potential source in patients presenting with distal emboli, which is almost always an indication for AAA repair. Infrequently a patient will present with complaints of a pulsatile mass and, rarely, large AAAs can cause symptomatic compression of surrounding structures, e.g., early satiety from duodenal compression and venous thrombosis from iliocaval compression. Chronic back and abdominal pain may be a presenting symptom of AAA that is ill defined and difficult to attribute directly to the aneurysm itself.

Etiology

- *Degenerative* are the most commonly encountered, noniatrogenic aneurysms.
- *Inflammatory* aneurysms are characterized by a fibrotic process in the retroperitoneum that involves the aneurysm as well as surrounding structures. All aneurysms may lie across a spectrum of inflammation.
- *Infectious or mycotic* aneurysms may be due to primary or secondary infection. Infection resulting in disrupted suture anastomoses can lead to the formation of pseudoaneurysms.
- *Postdissection* dilatation can occur from degeneration of the false lumen of a dissection as well as from any underlying pathology responsible for the dissection itself, e.g., Marfan's syndrome or Ehlers-Danlos syndromes.
- *Traumatic*

Diagnosis

Physical Exam

Physical exam varies depending upon the AAA size, obesity of the patient, and the skill and focus of the examiner and examination respectively. In general, the larger the AAA, the more likely it will be appreciated on abdominal examination. AAA may be falsely suspected in thin patients, patients with hypertension, tortuous aortas, and in patients with unrelated abdominal masses overlying the aorta.

Laboratory

Laboratory tests outside of vascular lab and other imaging modalities are utilized more in the preoperative work-up of the patient rather than in diagnosis of the aneurysm.

Imaging

1. *Ultrasound* is the most frequently used, least expensive, and least invasive modality. It is best utilized to diagnose and monitor AAAs until repair is considered. Ultrasound tends to underestimate diameter, have interobserver variability, and have difficulty visualizing the mesenteric aorta as well as iliac arteries [1]. More advanced imaging is used for preoperative evaluation and planning. Lastly, bedside ultrasound in the emergency department provides a rapid assessment of patients with symptomatic or ruptured AAA. *Sensitivity and specificity are high* in identification of AAA. Fluid collections are easily identified, but visualization of this is not specific for rupture.

    Screening with duplex ultrasound is recommended in males 65–75 years old who have a lifetime consumption of at least 100 cigarettes. The U.S. Preventative Services Task Force provided these recommendations in 1996 with an update in 2005 based upon several randomized and non-randomized studies. One such was the Multicentre Aneurysm Screening Study (MASS) trial which involved >70,000 men aged 65–74 and most notably demonstrated a 32 % reduction in AAA-related mortality [2].

2. *CT scan* provides more accurate AAA measurement but exposes the patient to radiation and IV contrast. There is less interobserver variability but some overestimation of tortuous aneurysms when measured obliquely and without

the assistance of centerline postprocessing software. CT angiography (CTA) is essential for preoperative planning of asymptomatic and symptomatic but stable patients alike. Furthermore, CT scan is the most accurate method of diagnosing ruptured AAA.

3. *Magnetic resonance imaging (MRI)* also provides more information than ultrasound and avoids the ionizing radiation of CT scan. However, it has issues related to cost, spatial resolution, nephrogenic sclerosis with gadolinium in patients with renal insufficiency, patient claustrophobia, and difficultly identifying calcifications. The continued improvement and accessibility of CTA relegates MRI/MRA to a secondary role in the evaluation of AAA.

4. *Angiography* was once standard in the preoperative evaluation of the AAA patient. However, given the quality of CTA and the information obtained with image postprocessing and reconstruction of the entire aorta anatomy, not just the flow lumen, angiography is now used only for specific perioperative needs, e.g., renal artery stenting and selective injections to determine renal mass supply by specific vessels.

Management

With regard to asymptomatic AAA, the choice between observation and intervention, whether surgical repair or endovascular stent-grafting, should take into account the risk of AAA rupture during observation based on aneurysm size and rate of growth, the interventional or operative risk, and the patient's life expectancy, which includes a number of areas of assessment. Symptomatic AAAs, those that have become painful and tender but have not ruptured, are repaired in a semiurgent fashion while ruptured aneurysms are repaired emergently. Repair may be with stent-grafting or open surgery depending upon anatomy and resources.

Asymptomatic AAA

The primary factor influencing decision to intervene is maximum aneurysm diameter. Various studies from the 1960s established that AAA size is directly proportional to rupture risk and the risk increases sharply between 5 and 6 cm.

The *UK Small Aneurysm Trial* [3] and the *Aneurysm Detection and Management* (ADAM) study [4] both randomized patients with AAA 4 to ~5.5 cm to early surgery or surveillance. In both studies there was no survival difference after 4.5 years though >60 % of patients in the surveillance arm eventually underwent repair. In summary, these studies showed a lack of benefit of early surgery for small aneurysms (<5.5 cm) even if operative mortality is low. Rupture risk in patients undergoing surveillance was approximately 1 %/year.

The Comparison of surveillance versus Aortic Endografting for Small Aneurysm Repair (CAESAR) trial compared observation and endovascular aneurysm repair (EVAR) for AAA 4.1–5.4 cm. There was no clear advantage between early and delayed EVAR as mortality and rupture rates are low in both groups. However, within 3 years, 60 % of the surveillance group will grow to require repair and 20 % might lose feasibility for EVAR [5].

We use the following schedule for follow-up of patients with small AAA (men <5.5 cm, women <5.0 cm) provided there is patient suitability for the operating room or interventional suite and a slow rate of growth <0.4 cm/6 months. For men with AAA <4.5 cm, duplex or CTA is performed with clinic visit every year; AAA 4.5–4.9 cm, duplex or CTA with clinic visit every 6 months; AAA 5.0–5.4 cm, duplex or CTA with clinic visit every 3 months. For women with AAA <4.0 cm, duplex or CTA is performed with clinic visit every year; AAA 4.0–4.4 cm, duplex or CTA with clinic visit every 6 months; AAA 4.5–4.9 cm, duplex or CTA with clinic visit every 3 months. During the observation period, best medical therapy is instituted, which consists of smoking cessation, exercise, aspirin, statin therapy, and consideration of ACE inhibitors and beta-blockers.

In consideration of EVAR versus open repair given suitable anatomy for either approach, patient age, comorbidities, compliance with medical advice, and functional status all play a major role in decision making. The EVAR-1 trial showed a lower 30-day mortality for EVAR over open repair (1.6 % versus 4.6 %) and a higher rate of secondary interventions for EVAR [6]. There was a reduction of aneurysm-related death at 4 years but similar all-cause mortalities at 2 years between the two groups. The Dutch Randomized Endovascular Aneurysm Management (DREAM) trial was smaller but showed similar results [7].

The OVER Veterans Affairs Cooperative Study Group randomly assigned patients with >5 cm AAA, who were candidates both endovascular or open repair, to each of these groups. The reduction in perioperative mortality (0.5 % endovascular versus 3 % open) was sustained at 3 years postop. However, there were six aneurysm ruptures in the endovascular group while there were none in the open group. Interestingly, survival was increased among patients under 70 years old in the endovascular group. The authors concluded that while survival advantage in the endovascular repair was sustained for several years, rupture in this group remained a concern. Furthermore, they concluded that endovascular repair did not lead to increased long-term survival as expected among older patients [8].

Symptomatic AAA

Irrespective of size, any aneurysm determined to be the cause of patient's pain or found to be tender on examination is deemed symptomatic and repaired in a semiurgent fashion due to its likely rapid growth and impending rupture. Inflamed and mycotic aneurysms also fall into this category. Aneurysms determined to be the source of thromboemboli are considered symptomatic as well and are repaired once the resultant ischemia is alleviated or during such procedures if the aneurysm can be treated with relative ease.

Ruptured AAA

The mortality of patients with ruptured AAA who arrive alive at the hospital is approximately 50 %. This has remained relatively unchanged for more than 50 years.

Transfer to an appropriate institution where definitive management can be carried out is the first priority. Usually there is ample time to acquire a stat CT angiography scan as well as transfer the patient to a higher level of care if necessary [9]. Reflection on the patient's prerupture functional status should also play into the decision to proceed with a highly morbid repair, which carries significant mortality.

The next and often concurrent consideration is appropriate resuscitation of the hypotensive patient. If resuscitation is aggressive, the resultant elevated blood pressure can overcome the stabilizing tamponade. This can lead to further hemorrhage and rapid decompensation prior to definitive therapy. Permissive hypotension [10], allowing the patient with a ruptured abdominal aortic aneurysm to maintain a systolic blood pressure of ~80–90 mmHg, is preferred so long as the patient displays appropriate mentation and maintains systemic and peripheral perfusion. This approach allows for temporary stabilization of the patient and time to obtain a CTA and formulate a plan of approach to repair. Additionally, hospital resources and surgeon expertise will influence the plan.

Blood should be cross matched as soon as possible with minimal threshold to activate the hospital's mass transfusion protocol with all products, i.e., plasma, platelets, cryoprecipitate, etc. Large bore IV access, an arterial line, and a Foley catheter all should be placed in the operating room. Red blood cell salvage via autotransfusion should be used for operating room suction. Consideration should be given to prepping and draping the patient awake before anesthesia as well as to using local anesthesia and sedation for EVAR in these circumstances of rupture.

Repair

1. *Open Surgery*. For the hemodynamically unstable patient, an open surgical approach, usually transperitoneal, in certain settings might be the most expeditious means of obtaining control of the aorta proximal to the rupture and stabilizing the hemorrhaging patient. This is often the best available approach for patients with inappropriate neck or access vessel anatomy for commercially available stent-grafts.

2. *EVAR*. In an era of abundant endovascular operating room suites and endovascular surgeon skill, nearly the only contraindication to EVAR for ruptured AAA is anatomic suitability. An occlusive balloon in the thoracic aorta can be achieved rapidly and might also be used for more rapid aortic control even if an open repair is ultimately performed. Postoperative complications include colon ischemia, multiorgan system failure, and continued hemorrhage sometimes due to type 2 endoleaks. In addition, renal failure, arterial ischemia, wound infection, and abdominal compartment syndrome, related to the hematoma, are further concerns. Drainage of the hematoma with or without management of the patient with an open abdomen is sometimes necessary. These complications are similar to those after open repair.

Follow-Up

Normal saline at 200 cc/h is infused for the first 12 h postop and then turned off to avoid overly aggressive crystalloid resuscitation. Bladder pressures are obtained if there is any suspicion of abdominal compartment syndrome. Blood products are given as needed. All organ systems are supported via usual ICU care.

After patient discharge from the hospital, all patients are seen in clinic at 4 weeks postoperatively. Little follow-up imaging is needed for patients after open repair of AAA unless otherwise indicated by symptoms or for known aneurysmal disease in other locations of the aorta or peripheral arteries.

For patients treated with EVAR, our practice has been to obtain CTA at the 4-week postoperative visit as well as at the 1-year visit. Type 2 endoleak is present in approximately 30 % of patients at 1 month and this reduces to 15 % at 4 months. Sac expansion and rupture only occur in 2–3 % of these patients. It is for this, as well as graft migration and aneurysmal degeneration of the EVAR landing zones, that continued imaging and lifetime follow-up of these patients are imperative. The schedule of CTA changes based upon the presence or absence of type 2 endoleak as well as that of aneurysm sac expansion. Treatment of type 2 endoleaks is reserved for those in which there is sac expansion. This is accomplished by IMA embolization from the SMA via the arc of Riolan or translumbar embolization, particularly if lumbar arteries are determined to be the culprit and there is no sac access from the IMA. Duplex ultrasound performed as an additional means of imaging observation of stent-grafts after the 1-year postoperative visit to reduce the number of CTAs performed per patient. CTA then can be repeated as needed during this long-term follow up period.

References

1. Lederle FA, Wilson SE, Johnson GR, Reinke DB, Littooy FN, Acher CW, et al. Variability in measurement of abdominal aortic aneurysms. Abdominal Aortic Aneurysm Detection and Management Veterans Administration Cooperative Study Group. J Vasc Surg. 1995;21(6):945–52.
2. Ashton HA, Buxton MJ, Day NE, Kim LG, Marteau TM, Scott RA, et al. the Multicentre Aneurysm Screening Study Group. The Multicentre Aneurysm Screening Study (MASS) into the effect of abdominal aortic aneurysm screening on mortality in men: a randomised controlled trial. Lancet. 2002; 360(9345):1531–9.

3. Powell JT, Brown LC, Forbes JF, Fowkes FG, Greenhalgh RM, Ruckley CV, et al. Final 12-year follow-up of surgery versus surveillance in the UK Small Aneurysm Trial. Br J Surg. 2007; 94(6):702–8.

4. Lederle FA, Johnson GR, Wilson SE, Chute EP, Hye RJ, Makaroun MS, et al. The aneurysm detection and management study screening program: validation cohort and final results. Aneurysm Detection and Management Veterans Affairs Cooperative Study Investigators. Arch Intern Med. 2000;160(10): 1425–30.

5. Cao P, De Rango P, Verzini F, Parlani G, Romano L, Cieri E, CAESAR Trial Group. Comparison of surveillance versus aortic endografting for small aneurysm repair (CAESAR): results from a randomised trial. Eur J Vasc Endovasc Surg. 2011; 41(1):13–25.

6. EVAR trial participants. Endovascular aneurysm repair versus open repair in patients with abdominal aortic aneurysm (EVAR trial 1): randomised controlled trial. Lancet. 2005; 365(9478):2179–86.

7. Prinssen M, Verhoeven EL, Buth J, Cuypers PW, van Sambeek MR, Balm R, Dutch Randomized Endovascular Aneurysm Management (DREAM) Trial Group, et al. A randomized trial comparing conventional and endovascular repair of abdominal aortic aneurysms. N Engl J Med. 2004;351(16):1607–18.

8. Lederle FA, Freischlag JA, Kyriakides TC, Matsumura JS, Padberg FT, Jr., Kohler TR, Kougias P, Jean-Claude JM, Cikrit DF, Swanson KM. Long-term comparison of endovascular and open repair of abdominal aortic aneurysm. The OVER Veterans Affairs Cooperative Study Group. N Engl J Med. 2012; 367:1988–1997. DOI:10.1056/NEJMoa1207481.

9. Lloyd GM, Bown MJ, Norwood MG, Deb R, Fishwick G, Bell PR, Sayers RD. Feasibility of preoperative computer tomography in patients with ruptured abdominal aortic aneurysm: a time-to-death study in patients without operation. J Vasc Surg. 2004;39(4):788–91.

10. Roberts K, Revell M, Youssef H, Bradbury AW, Adam DJ. Hypotensive resuscitation in patients with ruptured abdominal aortic aneurysm. Eur J Vasc Endovasc Surg. 2006;31(4):339–44.

Chapter 2
Acute Lower Limb Ischemia

Ramyar Gilani

Acute Limb Ischemia

Acute limb ischemia (ALI) of the lower extremities remains a challenging clinical dilemma despite recent advances in perioperative care, pharmacology, and technology. ALI can be defined as a decrease in limb arterial perfusion occurring within 14 days such that limb viability is threatened. Embolic and thrombotic phenomena constitute the majority of etiologies. The keys to successful outcomes include rapid and accurate diagnosis followed by expeditious intervention to restore limb perfusion.

Pathophysiology

The final common pathway for ALI is hypoperfusion and hypoxemia at the tissue level. Progression leads to cells' inability to regulate the environment and buildup of toxic radicals. Increased capillary permeability leads to swelling

R. Gilani, M.D. (✉)
Division of Vascular Surgery, Baylor College of Medicine,
1504 Taub Loop, Houston, TX 77030, USA

Michael E. DeBakey Department of Surgery, Baylor College of
Medicine, 1504 Taub Loop, Houston, TX 77030, USA
e-mail: rgilani@bcm.edu

S.K. Shah and D.G. Clair (eds.), *Cleveland Clinic Manual*
of Vascular Surgery, DOI 10.1007/978-1-4939-1631-3_2,
© Springer Science+Business Media New York 2014

first at the cellular level and can progress to increased pressures within the entire ischemic bed causing clinically significant compartment syndrome. Continued hypoxemia ultimately leads to cellular death, particularly within muscle and nervous tissue. Severe hypoperfusion and hypoxemia can lead to such changes within hours of insult. *Causative mechanisms* triggering the sequence of events involved in ALI are several but are predominately embolic or thrombotic in nature. Although the resulting sequelae are similar there are important distinctions to note between embolic and thrombotic events.

Embolism

Cardiac emboli secondary to atrial fibrillation, ventricular dysfunction, or valvular disease account for up to 90 % of embolic cases. However, other significant sources of emboli should be considered, such as more proximal atherosclerotic plaque and arterial aneurysm. Regardless of its source, the embolus will migrate to a point at which the vessel lumen becomes too small for further movement, causing vessel occlusion and blood stasis. This typically occurs at branch points such as the aortic, common femoral, or popliteal artery bifurcations. With stasis comes thrombus formation and propagation proximally and distally. This sequence of events occurs in a short period of time; therefore the onset of symptoms is rapid. The rapidity of onset also leaves insufficient time to generate collaterals and the degree of ischemia becomes severe.

Thrombosis

Thrombotic pathophysiology is initially an in situ process, commonly secondary to worsening native atherosclerotic burden or intimal hyperplasia initiated by prior interventions. These rather insidious processes lead to significant stenosis or occlusion over a longer period of time. However, a critical lesion will result in similar stasis and thrombus formation as with embolic etiology. This time course allows for the recruitment of collaterals to provide some degree of distal perfusion in the setting of thrombosis and therefore a more gradual onset of symptoms as well as lesser degree of ischemia distally. However, if thrombosis continues to a point where collaterals are also involved or lacking severe ischemia will result.

Diagnosis

History and Examination

The diagnosis of ALI is made clinically and should include determination of the etiology and degree of ischemia. Diagnosis can be made readily through history, physical exam, and use of a handheld Doppler.

- Determination of limb ischemia is classically investigated through the application of the "5 Ps": pulselessness, pain, pallor, paresthesia, and paralysis—occurring in that order. A sixth "P," poikilothermia, is sometimes added and is an ominous sign. While obtaining history, attention should be given to onset, location, and severity of pain, prior history of claudication or interventions, risk factors for atherosclerosis, and any history suggesting embolic phenomenon.
- As mentioned before, embolic events produce severe symptoms rather quickly whereas thrombotic pathology can be more gradual. History of claudication or vascular intervention particularly in the setting of risk factors tends to be suggestive of thrombosis.
- Physical examination should include a complete pulse exam as well as attention to cardiac rhythm and the possible presence of aneurysmal disease (aortic, femoral, and popliteal). The presence of normal pulses, an aneurysm, or cardiac arrhythmia is suggestive of embolic disease. The level at which a pulse or signal is no longer appreciated aids in determining the location of pathology. Provocative maneuvers such as elevation and lowering can serve to intensify and alleviate symptoms respectively in ALI.

TABLE 2.1. Rutherford classification of acute limb ischemia.

Class	Need for intervention	Examination	Arterial signal	Venous signal
I	Limb not threatened; elective intervention	No sensorimotor deficits	+	+
IIa	Limb threatened; urgent intervention	Mild sensory loss at most; no motor signs	−	+
IIb	Limb threatened; emergent intervention	Sensory loss, possible rest pain. Mild weakness	−	+
III	Limb irreversibly damaged	Profound sensorimotor loss	−	−

- Determining the degree of ischemia is clinically useful as a guide for timing of appropriate intervention. The Rutherford classification [1] (Table 2.1) serves as a reference for categorizing degrees of severity in ALI. This grading scale is intended to be applicable at the bedside through physical exam and use of a handheld Doppler. After applying categorization, recommendations are provided for the appropriate management (Table 2.1).

Imaging

Once a diagnosis of ALI has been formulated, further characterization of arterial anatomy and status is best evaluated through diagnostic imaging. The predominating imaging modalities utilized in this assessment are computed tomographic angiography (CTA) and traditional contrast angiography with some limited role for duplex ultrasound:

- *CTA* is being increasingly used as the preferred initial imaging exam for ALI due to several attributes. Due to systemic delivery of contrast, CTA can effectively delineate entire limb arterial anatomy simultaneously. This is useful for identifying the extent of thrombosis as well as proximal and distal vessel targets for intervention. Sluggish flow particularly within the tibial vessels and distally can limit the delivery of contrast and therefore reduce the amount of information provided by the exam. Additional information readily available via CTA includes vessel calcification, vessel diameter, collateralization, and presence of previous stents or bypass grafts. CTA is, however, a static study providing very little information about flow dynamics. Disadvantages include the need for radiation and potentially nephrotoxic contrast.

- *Contrast angiography* is considered by many to be the gold-standard imaging modality for ALI. Angiography has the indisputable advantage of being both diagnostic and potentially therapeutic. It also provides information regarding flow characteristics. Angiography, however, only provides information available through opacification of the vessel lumen and therefore does not provide any extralumenal assessment. Collateral pathways can be quite variable in ALI and the ability to opacify vessels distal to the affected region requires catheter selection of the appropriate supplying collateral pathway as well as adequate timing to allow for contrast to be delivered. Angiography, like CTA, also uses radiation and potentially nephrotoxic contrast; however, contrast volumes are often less than CTA. Additional risks are associated with arterial cannulation and intralumenal manipulation but are relatively minimal.
- *Duplex ultrasound* (US), although not frequently used for ALI, can provide some valuable information expeditiously, especially if readily performed by the provider. In cases of strongly suspected arterial embolism, the location of embolus can be quickly confirmed via US. Also potential access points for arterial cannulation can be quickly assessed for feasibility. Lastly, availability of venous conduit for arterial reconstruction can be ascertained.

Treatment

Once a diagnosis of ALI has been established, appropriate further management should be expeditiously applied. Treatment strategies can be divided into two arms: *anticoagulation and revascularization.* Early anticoagulation via systemic

TABLE 2.2.   Contraindication to thrombolysis.

Relative	Systolic BP > 180 mmHg; diastolic BP > 110 mmHg
	Recent major surgery, including eye surgery
	Pregnancy
	Trauma within 10 days
	Hepatic failure
	Bacterial endocarditis
Absolute	GI bleeding within 10 days
	Intracranial or spinal surgery within 3 months
	Head injury within 3 months
	Stroke within 6 months

heparinization is the initial management maneuver in cases of ALI as long as no contraindication to anticoagulation exists (Table 2.2). Revascularization strategies consist of endovascular techniques, open surgical revascularization, and hybrid procedures. All of the different treatment modalities for ALI are not intended to be competitive but rather complimentary. The astute clinician should be proficient with all and be prepared to apply them to the specific scenario on hand:

- Management of Rutherford Class I ischemia with anticoagulation alone is appropriate, allowing time for more thorough evaluation and possibly elective revascularization.
- For Class IIa and IIb ischemia, anticoagulation alone is not sufficient and prompt revascularization is warranted to prevent further ischemic damage.
- Class III ischemia implies irreversible damage requiring some level of amputation; however, treatment may be incorporated to lower the level of amputation.

Anticoagulation

Anticoagulation through systemic heparinization serves several purposes. Most importantly, risk of further clot propagation is decreased especially in small distal runoff vessels where flow can become quite static. Second, in the cases of embolism, risk of recurrent embolism can be reduced. Lastly, through antiinflammatory and microcirculation properties, heparin may improve symptomatology and even restore some perfusion such that more time for further evaluation is allowed. Low molecular-weight heparin serves no role in the initial management of ALI.

Catheter-Directed Thrombolysis

The basis for catheter-directed thrombolysis (CDT) is the delivery of a thrombolytic agent via an infusion catheter directly into the site of thrombus, thereby increasing the local concentration of agent and reducing systemic exposure. The most common agents encountered in the literature are urokinase (UK) and tissue plasminogen activator (t-PA). Because thrombolysis is a function of an enzymatic reaction, time is required to produce demonstrable clot resolution, which is an important consideration in cases of advanced ischemia. However, CDT has the very important and distinct ability to achieve clot resolution within distal outflow vessels that would not be resolved with other techniques. The efficacy of CDT and its variations have been validated through clinical trials, of which the three most prominent include the Rochester study, Surgery versus Thrombolysis for Ischemia of the Lower Extremity (STILE), and Thrombolysis Or Peripheral Arterial Surgery (TOPAS) [2–4].

Technique

There are technical considerations for CDT to enhance success and mitigate complications. Point of access is selected at a remote site away from the affected region, most commonly the contralateral common femoral or brachial artery. This serves to prevent thrombolytic agent from interfering with the access site. Therefore, it is important to know the patency of the potential access vessels. Access via the brachial artery limits the ability to deliver larger profile devices and additional access point may be later required to perform further interventions after successful clot resolution. Cannulation should be performed with ultrasound guidance to ensure success with the first attempt to limit potential sources of bleeding. Once access is established, the critical maneuver of traversing the thrombosed region is performed. The desired target outflow vessel can be identified via prior CTA or angiography. After crossing, cannulation of the true lumen should be confirmed with an angiogram. Next, a drug delivery device is positioned to infuse agent from a point immediately proximal to the area of thrombus including the thrombosed region up to a point just distal to the thrombus within the outflow vessel. Infusion catheters are typically used in aorto-iliac and femoro-popliteal segments, whereas infusion wires are more appropriate for tibial infusions. In long segment occlusions, a combination of catheter and wire is required connected with a Tuohy-Borst adapter. There is some evidence that the use of ultrasound enhanced infusion catheters (EKOS Corp., Bothell, WA) may expedite thrombolysis particularly in thrombosed grafts and may be considered for use. After securing the infusion apparatus in proper position, infusion of thrombolytic agent commences. A bolus of 5 mg tPA into the system to acutely increase agent concentration is acceptable. Infusion of the agent is continued at a rate of 0.5–1.0 mg/h continued over 12–24 h. After this period, repeat angiography is performed to assess progress and perform adjustments. The goal of CDT is to lyse acute thrombus within the occluded segment and reveal the so-called "culprit" lesion instigating the thrombosis. Identifying and appropriately treating the "culprit" lesion is predictive of durable success. Furthermore, sufficient outflow into the distal limb must also be established to provide success. It is important to note that t-PA requires fibrin rich clot in order to be effective. In cases of embolism, where the thromboembolism may be more chronic in nature, t-PA can be less efficacious in clot resolution and alternative open interventional strategies may be more effective. Also with the potential for systemic fibrinolysis, dissolution of residual thrombus at the source poses the risk for additional embolic events with serious consequences such as cerebrovascular events.

Percutaneous Mechanical Thrombectomy

Percutaneous mechanical thrombectomy (PMT) functions to rapidly decrease thrombus burden and restore a flow lumen establishing some degree of in-line distal perfusion, thereby decreasing the delay required for CDT. A wide variety of devices are available to perform PMT but all perform either by direct aspiration or emulsification and extraction of thrombus.

Technique

PMT is technically performed initially in a similar fashion as CDT requiring appropriate arterial access and wire traversal of the thrombosed vessel. Direct aspiration of thrombus is performed via sheath aspiration or specifically designed aspiration catheters. With sheath aspiration, the largest allowable sheath is positioned within the thrombus and, while aspirating, slowly withdrawn to extract thrombus into the sheath. With each pass the sheath must be completely withdrawn and the lumen flushed prior to attempting another pass. Alternatively, an aspiration catheter can be used in a similar fashion. These devices are typically lower profile than an effectively sized aspiration sheath and do not require loss of sheath access. Aspiration of fragmented thrombus, also known as rheolytic thrombectomy (RT), is an alternative to direct thrombus aspiration.

Commonly used devices for RT are the Angiojet system (Possis Medical Inc., Minneapolis, MN) and the Trellis system (Covidien, Manchester, MA). The Angiojet design applies the Bernoulli principle by using a high pressure high velocity jet of solution within a flow channel creating a vacuum effect through adjacently placed side holes. As the catheter is passed through the thrombus, the jet is activated and clot is fragmented and aspirated. Additional t-PA can be mixed into the solution and introduced into the fragmented thrombus via the "power pulse spray" technique. This provides the theoretical advantage of exposing more thrombus surface area to the lytic agent. Attention must be given to the amount of solution used as increasing amounts are associated with hemolysis and renal dysfunction. As clot fragmentation occurs, the risk of further thromboembolism is present. The Trellis system functions by isolating a thrombosed segment of vessel between proximal and distal inflated balloons. Within this segment a wire is present and when activated oscillates in a sinusoidal fashion causing mechanical fragmentation. The resulting fragmented clot is then aspirated before deflating the balloons, reducing the risk of additional thromboembolism; however, this risk is not eliminated. As with the Angiojet, the Trellis allows for introduction of lytic agent into the fragmented thrombus. After allowing sufficient time for thrombolysis, the t-PA can be aspirated which reduces the risk of systemic fibrinolysis.

Open Revascularization

Despite the tremendous expansion and application of endovascular techniques to ALI, open revascularization via thromboembolectomy, endarterectomy, and bypass continues to have a significant role in the management of ALI. Unfortunately, open interventions have been associated with mortality rates of 20–30 % [5, 6]. However, the major trials comparing open surgery to thrombolysis have failed to demonstrate superiority and therefore consensus has never been agreed upon. Nevertheless, in properly and appropriately selected scenarios such as embolism or advanced severe ischemia, open surgery remains effective first-line therapy. Many procedures can be performed with local or regional anesthesia but more involved interventions may require general anesthesia.

Technical Considerations

Although relatively simple to conceive, there are some key technical aspects to consider when performing thromboembolectomy. It is helpful to know beforehand if embolism or native thrombosis is suspected. If this is unknown, palpation of the artery of interest revealing normal vessel wall tends to favor embolism. On the other hand, a calcified hard vessel is suggestive of thrombosis. This important distinction determines the orientation of the arteriotomy performed: a transverse incision for an embolism and a longitudinal one for thrombosis allowing for endarterectomy. The transverse arteriotomy should be placed in proximity of a vessel bifurcation to allow direction and passage of balloon catheters distally into each branch vessel. For example, when performing a common femoral artery embolectomy, the arteriotomy is made just proximal to the bifurcation to allow for passage of balloon catheters into the deep femoral and superficial femoral arteries. Of course, balloon catheters are also passed proximally through the inflow source. Despite the clinical efficacy, however, considerable residual thrombus can remain within the distal arterial bed even after the best attempts with balloon catheters. Completion angiography is therefore strongly suggested.

Open vascular reconstruction via *thromboendarterectomy* and *surgical bypass* is not to be forgotten for ALI management. They serve to restore perfusion rapidly with durable results albeit via more invasive procedures. These procedures are performed for ALI as in other settings with regard to inflow, outflow, and conduit selection. Adjunct procedures such as stenting for a proximal iliac lesion or local thrombolysis for a thrombosed popliteal artery aneurysm may be added in the course of open reconstruction.

Complications

Complications relating to ALI and its management can be categorized into the following: limb related, procedural related, and organ-system related. Patients typically have preexisting comorbidities and therefore are already at some increased risk for complications. Close observation within a monitored clinical setting with attention to detail and appropriate treatment selection are the best methods for mitigating complications in the perioperative setting.

Limb Loss

Limb loss is a real possibility with ALI even in the setting of a successful procedural outcome. Furthermore, delay in treatment may ultimately keep a limb viable but dysfunctional secondary to nerve or muscle injury. Revascularized limbs are at risk for developing severe edema and secondary compartment syndrome. Limbs noted to have increasing pressures clinically or via compartment pressure measurement (>30 mmHg) should undergo immediate *fasciotomy*.

Procedural Risks

Performing endovascular and open procedures always carries a certain level of risk for standard procedural complications such as bleeding, hematoma, infection, poor wound healing, etc., and is no different in the setting of ALI. However, *severe bleeding complications* (10 %) of a different variety are a potential complication with exposure to thrombolytic agent, particularly noncompressible hemorrhage. Bleeding into the central nervous system (CNS), gastrointestinal (GI) tract, eye, or body cavity can have serious consequences, with CNS bleeds (1–2 %) being the most devastating. Careful questioning with regard to recent surgery especially within the CNS, recent stroke, recent trauma, history of bleeding, malignancy, and any other condition to be complicated by systemic fibrinolysis should be elucidated. During ongoing thrombolysis, continuous laboratory evaluation of coagulation including PT, PTT, INR, fibrinogen, and CBC should be performed. Evidence of *systemic fibrinolysis* or bleeding should prompt cessation of thrombolytic therapy. Also close monitoring of arterial blood pressure and aggressive treatment of hypertension is good practice.

Organ-System Complications

Given the degree of comorbidity in ALI patients, it is not surprising that cardiopulmonary complications of myocardial infarction, congestive heart failure exacerbation, and pulmonary failure remain real threats to desirable outcomes. What is less intuitive is the effect of revascularization on the cardiopulmonary system. When an ischemic limb becomes revascularized, the accumulated toxins and metabolites become systemic with potential deleterious effects such as cardiac arrhythmias and shock. Treatment is purely supportive; however, anticipation of these outcomes can initiate preparedness and therapy prior to occurrence. Significant degrees of muscle necrosis can lead to *myoglobinemia* that has negative consequences on renal function. Although significant permanent renal dysfunction can be usually avoided with appropriate supportive care, severe continuous myoglobinemia can precipitate permanent renal dysfunction forcing the decision of life over limb.

References

1. Rutherford RB, Baker JD, Ernst C, Johnston KW, Porter JM, Ahn S, Jones DN. Recommended standards for reports dealing with lower extremity ischemia: revised version. J Vasc Surg. 1997;26(3):517–38.
2. Ouriel K, Shortell CK, DeWeese JA, Green RM, Francis CW, Azodo MV, Gutierrez OH, Manzione JV, Cox C, Marder VJ. A comparison of thrombolytic therapy with operative revascularization in the initial treatment of acute peripheral arterial ischemia. J Vasc Surg. 1994;19(6):1021–30.
3. Results of a prospective randomized trial evaluating surgery versus thrombolysis for ischemia of the lower extremity. The STILE trial. Ann Surg. 1994; 220(3):251–66, discussion 266–8.
4. Ouriel K, Veith FJ, Sasahara AA. A comparison of recombinant urokinase with vascular surgery as initial treatment for acute arterial occlusion of the legs. Thrombolysis or Peripheral Arterial Surgery (TOPAS) Investigators. N Engl J Med. 1998;338(16): 1105–11.
5. Blaisdell FW, Steele M, Allen RE. Management of acute lower extremity arterial ischemia due to embolism and thrombosis. Surgery. 1978;84(6):822–34.
6. Jivegård L, Holm J, Scherstén T. Acute limb ischemia due to arterial embolism or thrombosis: influence of limb ischemia versus pre-existing cardiac disease on postoperative mortality rate. J Cardiovasc Surg (Torino). 1988;29(1):32–6.

Chapter 3
Aortoiliac Disease

Julie E. Adams

Introduction

Patients with peripheral arterial disease commonly present with symptoms of arterial claudication, rest pain, or with evidence of tissue loss. Arterial disease can be present at multiple levels, but the careful evaluation of the aortoiliac segment is an important component of the initial approach to the patient with chronic limb ischemia.

Clinical Presentation

Aortoiliac segment, or inflow, disease is a common cause of chronic lower limb ischemia. Patients may present along a spectrum of symptom severity. Mildly affected patients may report typical symptoms of lower extremity claudication such as pain with ambulation, worse when walking up an incline, and relieved by rest. Although many patients may only describe calf symptoms, a clue to the presence of aortoiliac segment disease may be the description of crampy pain in the

J.E. Adams, M.D. (✉)
Department of Surgery, Fletcher Allen Health Care,
111 Colchester Ave., Burlington, VT 05401, USA
e-mail: julie.adams@vtmednet.org

S.K. Shah and D.G. Clair (eds.), *Cleveland Clinic Manual of Vascular Surgery*, DOI 10.1007/978-1-4939-1631-3_3,
© Springer Science+Business Media New York 2014

buttocks or thighs and not just the calf muscle groups. Some men may report erectile dysfunction, which along with lower extremity claudication, leg muscle atrophy, and reduced femoral pulses comprise Leriche syndrome. Aortoiliac disease may progress to rest pain, nonhealing ulcers, or gangrene of the feet. This may be secondary to multilevel disease, inadequacy of collaterals, or distal embolization from shaggy atherosclerotic plaque in the aortoiliac segment.

Blue toe syndrome is a specific clinical presentation that can occur from disease in the aortoiliac segment. Mural aortic thrombus or shaggy atheromatous plaque in any segment of the aorta or iliac arteries can be an embolic source. Patients present with bilateral painful bluish discoloration of the toes and usually palpable pedal pulses.

Pathology

The anatomic spectrum of aortoiliac occlusive disease has been well-defined in the vascular literature. The TransAtlantic Inter-Society Consensus (TASC) recommendations were most recently updated in 2007 (Table 3.1) [1]. Initially TASC A and B lesions have been treated by endovascular means and TASC C and D lesions by surgical revascularization.

There is a subset of patients with aortoiliac occlusive disease who have small arteries, the so-called *hypoplastic aortoiliac syndrome*. This typically affects younger women with associated atherosclerotic disease [2].

Diagnosis

Physical Examination

Physical examination can be very helpful in localizing disease in patients with symptomatic lower extremity occlusive disease. The absence of normal femoral pulses indicates an inflow stenosis or occlusion. Bilaterally diminished femoral

TABLE 3.1. TASC II classification of aortoiliac disease.

A
- Stenosis of the CIA
- Unilateral or bilateral single ≤3 cm stenosis of EIA

B
- Single ≤3 cm stenosis of infrarenal aorta
- Unilateral CIA occlusion
- Unilateral single or multiple EIA stenoses with a total length of 3–10 cm without involvement of the CFA
- Unilateral EIA occlusion without IIA or CFA involvement

C
- Bilateral CIA occlusion
- Bilateral single or multiple EIA stenoses with a total length of 3–10 cm without involvement of the CFA
- Unilateral EIA stenosis extending into the CFA
- Unilateral EIA occlusion extending into the IIA or CFA
- Heavily calcified unilateral EIA occlusion

D
- Infrarenal aortoiliac occlusion
- Diffuse aortic and biiliac disease
- Multiple stenosis of the a unilateral CIA, EIA, CFA
- Unilateral CIA and EIA occlusion
- Bilateral EIA occlusion
- Iliac stenosis in patients with abdominal aortic aneurysm requiring open repair or other lesions demanding open aortic or iliac repair

pulses could indicate aortic and/or bilateral iliac occlusive disease while the presence of a normal femoral pulse on one side would point to a more severe unilateral iliac process. Palpation of pulses can sometimes be misleading, though, as some patients with significant aortoiliac occlusive disease may have such well-developed collaterals that a palpable pulse is present even distal to an occlusion. As with the initial evaluation of any patient with symptomatic PAD, a complete evaluation of upper and lower extremity pulses should occur routinely.

Inspection of the extremities for signs of tissue loss, dependent rubor, or concomitant venous disease is also part of a complete evaluation.

Imaging

Vascular Lab

1. *Segmental pressures* can provide objective evidence of disease in the inflow segment. A decrease in pressure of 20 mmHg or more between the brachial artery and the thigh cuffs would indicate a hemodynamically significant stenosis. This could be present unilaterally or bilaterally, offering a clue to distribution of disease. A segmental pressure study with additional reductions in pressure between the thigh and calf or ankle segments would indicate multi-level disease.

   A normal resting study does not rule out significant arterial stenosis, and the vascular lab technologist can exercise a patient with typical symptoms of claudication and a normal resting study to detect a drop in pressure [3].

2. *Arterial Duplex* can be a helpful adjunct in the initial evaluation of a patient with any lower extremity symptoms. Best performed while a patient is fasting, an aortoiliac duplex can often detect hemodynamically significant stenoses or occlusions. The presence of aneurysm or ectasia, complex atheromatous plaque, or mobile thrombus can also be detected as well as the presence of concomitant common femoral artery disease. This can be helpful information if one is contemplating invasive angiography for further diagnostic evaluation or intervention.

Computed Tomography Angiography

CT angiography can be diagnostic and greatly aid in treatment planning. The aortoiliac diameters, extent of calcification, and presence of mural thrombus or concomitant ectasia can help with choosing the best method of revascularization. This is often the preferred imaging test if one does not think an endovascular approach is indicated.

Angiography

Angiography is the preferred imaging test if endovascular intervention is planned, as it can be done at the same time as diagnostic imaging. A complete initial exam should include an abdominal aortogram with imaging of the aorta from renal arteries inferiorly and oblique views of the pelvis if required for visualization of disease relative to the origins of the hypogastric arteries. Bilateral runoff imaging should also be performed to the feet. This will both evaluate for concomitant infrainguinal disease and serve as a baseline to later assess for embolic complications of intervention that may require treatment.

Management

Direct Reconstruction

Aortobifemoral Bypass

Aortobifemoral bypass (ABF) has traditionally been considered the standard for the treatment of aortoiliac occlusive disease. Long-term patency rates have exceeded 75–90 %, depending on the series [4–6]. Age of patient has been well-established as inversely correlating with both primary and secondary patency [4, 6]. Five-year primary patency after ABF has been reported as 66 ± 8 % in patients younger than 50 years of age and as greater than 96 ± 2 % for those older than 60 years of age [6]. Use of autogenous superficial femoral vein as a conduit has been shown to augment the patency in this younger group of patients but at the expense of longer operating time and increased need for lower extremity fasciotomies [7]. Most surgeons choose either Dacron or ring-reinforced PTFE for conduit.

The *options for the proximal graft configuration* are an end-to-end or end-to-side aortic anastomosis. The classic situation where an end-to-side proximal anastomosis is routinely indicated involves a patient with bilateral external iliac artery occlusions and patent common iliac arteries. With this anatomy, perfusion of the hypogastric arteries is only possible with an end-to-side proximal anastomosis, preserving important pelvic blood flow. Situations where an end-to-end aortic anastomosis is preferable include patients with concomitant infrarenal aortic or iliac aneurysmal disease or atheromatous plaque or mural thrombus thought to be a source of peripheral embolization.

The *surgical approach* for aortobifemoral bypass generally involves making the femoral incisions first, either longitudinally or transversely. Once vascular control is obtained in the groins, the midline abdominal incision is made and the standard approach to the aorta is undertaken. There may be increased collaterals in the abdominal wall and retroperitoneum compared to a patient with aneurysmal pathology.

Each tunnel should be created by initially using one's fingers to gently create a plane just anterior to the iliac arteries, care being taken to avoid ureteral or venous injury. Once the tunnel is digitally created, an aortic clamp can be passed along one's hand to allow for placement of an umbilical tape through the tunnel on each side. The patient should be fully heparinized. In general, the aortic pathology extends close to the renal arteries, and so proximal control should be obtained close to the renal arteries. Separate vascular control of each renal artery with vessel loops may be required for protection against embolization. If there is thrombus extending to the renal orifices as seen in an aortic occlusion, suprarenal control should also be obtained and the suprarenal clamp briefly released to "flush" out the thrombus and allow for subsequent placement of the clamp more distally. In this situation an end-to-end anastomosis is appropriate. Distal control can often be obtained in the aorta itself and avoid dissection in the pelvis. Occasionally a sidebiting clamp can be applied to the aorta and obviate the need for two separate clamps. In a stiff, calcified aorta, a portion of aortic wall can be excised to allow for better visualization of the lumen.

After the proximal anastomosis is complete, the limbs of the graft are clamped separately and passed through each tunnel. Care is taken to avoid either excessive tension or redundancy when planning the distal anastomosis. If the superficial femoral artery (SFA) is patent, the common femoral arteriotomy should be directed onto the proximal SFA. If occluded, the graft can be directed onto the origin of the profunda, and profundaplasty effectively achieved. Prior to release of the clamps, copious flushing should occur to avoid distal embolization of any atheromatous material from the aorta. The retroperitoneal tissue can be reapproximated and the groins closed in multiple layers.

Aortoiliac Endarterectomy

Aortoiliac endarterectomy has become an uncommonly performed procedure for localized pathology in this anatomic region but has been shown to have comparable patency rates when compared to aortofemoral bypass or iliofemoral bypass. Patients with small vessels, where both endovascular and open interventions may pose some difficulty, may also benefit from endarterectomy. In addition to a lower mortality rate than aortofemoral bypass, endarterectomy also avoids the use of prosthestic material. Unfortunately many patients do not have focal areas of disease that would make them candidates for this operation [8] (Fig. 3.1a, b).

Extraanatomic Bypass

Extraanatomic bypass is widely accepted as inferior to direct reconstruction with regard to patency rates. It is, however, a viable option for patients medically unfit for initial or redo aortic surgery.

Axillofemoral Bypass

Axillofemoral bypass grafting can be performed in patients with either unilateral or bilateral chronic limb ischemia. For patients with planned bilateral lower extremity revascularization, the bypass generally originates from the right axillary artery and extends in a subcutaneous tunnel to the right

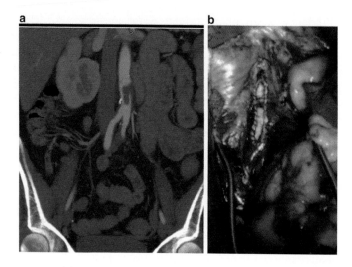

FIG. 3.1.   (**a**) Coronal reconstructions reveal a mural aortic thrombus associated with an underlying focal aortic atherosclerotic plaque. This failed to resolve with anticoagulation and caused bilateral lower extremity claudication. (**b**) Intraoperative photo now shows patient s/p aortic endarterectomy and patch angioplasty with bovine pericardium.

femoral artery where a distal anastomosis is performed, similar to that done in aortofemoral bypass. A second femorofemoral bypass is then performed to revascularize the left leg. Pre-bifurcated grafts that obviate the need for a graft–graft femoral anastomosis are commercially available. The left axillary artery can also be used as a source of inflow. Prior to choosing the inflow site, evaluation of the upper extremities for proximal subclavian stenoses should occur. For these operations, the patient's extremity, chest and abdomen, and lower extremities should be prepped and draped. The incision is infraclavicular, and the pectoralis minor muscle can be divided to allow access to the axillary artery. After tunneling the graft, it should be laid with a gentle C-shaped configuration to allow for full abduction of the arm without excessive tension at the proximal anastomosis, which should be on the medial aspect of the first portion of the axillary artery. Attention to detail in this portion of the procedure can decrease the risk of avulsion of the graft with subsequent vigorous abduction.

There is no consensus on the ideal *conduit*, but many surgeons continue to use externally reinforced polyester or PTFE because of theoretical concerns for extrinsic compression.

Alternative axillobifemoral bypass configurations involving interruptions of the ipsilateral common iliac artery are also sometimes used.

Femorofemoral Bypass

Femorofemoral bypass is an option for patients with unilateral iliac stenosis or occlusion who are not candidates for endovascular intervention or direct aortofemoral bypass. Becoming more common is the use of concomitant iliac stenting in the setting of femorofemoral bypass grafting [9]. This has unfortunately been associated with a decline in both primary and assisted primary graft patency. Huded et al. reported a 5-year primary patency of 44 % for patients undergoing inflow iliac PTA or stenting at time of femorofemoral bypass. During the same time period, patients undergoing axillofemoral bypass enjoyed a 74 % 5-year primary patency while those undergoing femorofemoral bypass without inflow stenting had a 71 % 5-year patency [9].

There has been no consistently demonstrated difference when using polyester, expanded PTFE, or externally reinforced PTFE.

There is no clear patency difference among conduit diameters ranging from 6 to 9 mm.

Thoracofemoral Bypass

Thoracofemoral bypass is a rarely performed procedure, indicated only when the abdominal aorta is unsuitable for use as an inflow source. This may be due to extensive prior abdominal aortic surgery, infection, or radiation [10].

Endovascular Therapy

Endovascular therapy for aortoiliac occlusive disease includes balloon angioplasty, placement of bare stents, or use of stent grafts. TASC classification has traditionally guided surgeons toward either open or endovascular therapy, though there are many reports of durable results with endovascular treatment of complex aortoiliac disease. Endovascular therapy is the accepted treatment for unilateral or bilateral stenoses of the common iliac arteries, unilateral or bilateral short ≤3 cm stenoses of the external iliac arteries, all considered TASC A lesions. It is also accepted for the treatment of TASC B lesions: short ≤3 cm stenoses of the infrarenal aorta, unilateral common iliac occlusions, single or multiple stenoses totaling 3–10 cm of the external iliac arteries or unilateral external iliac artery occlusions, the latter two not involving the internal iliac or common femoral arteries [1].

The *Dutch Iliac Stent Trial* randomized patients with intermittent claudication to primary stenting or primary angioplasty with selective stenting for bailout. Lesions were similar in the two groups. Selective stenting was found to be an acceptable approach to iliac interventions as the patency rates did not significantly differ at 1 year [11]. This study was limited by lack of long-term follow-up and absence of patients with critical limb ischemia.

More complex TASC C and D lesions may also be amenable to endovascular therapy, though many patients may also be candidates for surgical reconstruction. A series from the Cleveland Clinic published in 2006 revealed acceptable 3-year patency rates in patients with TASC B, C, and D chronic symptomatic iliac occlusions treated with endovascular therapy. Primary patency was similar in all groups at 76 %. Patients with TASC B and C lesions had secondary patency rates of 95 and 93 % while TASC D patients had secondary patency rates of 83 %, which did not reach statistical significance [12].

The use of covered stents has been studied with regard to patency for endovascular aortoiliac interventions. The *COvered versus Balloon Expandable Stent Trial* (*COBEST*) was the first randomized trial between bare and covered stents for the iliac arteries. The investigators found an improvement in patency for TASC C and D lesions compared with bare stents but not for TASC B lesions. In this trial, patients with hemodynamically significant dissections and recurrent stenoses after angioplasty were randomized to bare stents or balloon expandable PTFE covered stents. Patients with covered stents had fewer interventions for restenosis [13, 14].

Complications

Open surgical treatment for aortoiliac occlusive disease encompasses a wide range of complications. Patients undergoing major aortic surgery can often carry a higher risk of mortality, though many patients undergoing extraanatomic bypass may have risks that prohibit them from aortic surgery as an option. This sicker patient group with higher mortality is evident in the series published by Hertzer et al. in 2007 [4]. In this series, patients undergoing direct reconstruction carried an operative mortality rate of 2.3 % while patients undergoing axillofemoral bypass had a 12 % 30-day mortality rate [4]. This has been attributed to the concomitant medical problems that prohibited direct aortic reconstruction. This highlights the importance of patient selection when planning major aortic surgery.

Open surgery also carries with it the risks of cardiopulmonary complications, wound complications, graft thrombosis, and infection.

Endovascular interventions can have complications from either the access site or the target site. Patients also have the associated cardiovascular risks of anesthesia and sedation. *Access site complications* include bleeding, pseudoaneurysm formation, thrombosis, and dissection. Sometimes open surgery is urgently required to treat active hemorrhage or distal ischemia. The use of multiple access sites increases the opportunities for complications. At or from the target site of intervention there are reports of dissection and thrombosis, rupture, or distal embolization. *Device-related complications* could include stent migration, malpositioning, and incomplete expansion. Late complications often stem from restenosis of previously treated vessels [15, 16].

References

1. Norgren I, Hiatt WR, Dormandy JA, Nehler MR, Harris KA, Fowkes FGR. Inter-society consensus for the management of peripheral arterial disease (TASC II). J Vasc Surg. 2007;45(Suppl S): S5–67.
2. Walton B, Dougherty K, Mortazavi A, Strickman N, Krajcer Z. Percutaneous intervention for the treatment of hypoplastic aortoiliac syndrome. Catheter Cardiovasc Interv. 2003; 60(3):329–34.
3. Stein R, Hriljac I, Halperin J, Gustavson S, Teodorescu V, Olin J. Limitation of the resting ankle-brachial index in symptomatic patients with peripheral arterial disease. Vasc Med. 2006;11: 29–33.
4. Hertzer N, Bena J, Karafa M. A personal experience with direct reconstruction and extra-anatomic bypass for aortoiliofemoral occlusive disease. J Vasc Surg. 2007;45:527–35.
5. Szilagyi D, Elliott J, Smith R, Reddy D, McPharlin M. A thirty-year survey of reconstructive surgical treatment of aortoiliac occlusive disease. J Vasc Surg. 1986;3:421–36.
6. Reed A, Conte M, Donaldson M, Mannick J, Whittemore A, Belkin M. The impact of patient age and aortic size on the results of aortobifemoral bypass grafting. J Vasc Surg. 2003;37:1219–25.
7. Jackson M, Ali A, Bell C, Modrall JG, Welborn MB, Scoggins E, et al. Aortofemoral bypass in young patients with premature atherosclerosis: is superficial femoral vein superior to Dacron? J Vasc Surg. 2004;40:17–23.
8. Chiu K, Davies R, Nightingale P, Bradbury A, Adam D. Review of direct anatomical open surgical management of atherosclerotic aorto-iliac occlusive disease. Eur J Vasc Endovasc Surg. 2010;39:460–71.
9. Huded C, Goodney P, Powell R, Nolan B, Rzucidlo E, Simone S, et al. The impact of adjunctive iliac stenting on femoral-femoral bypass in contemporary practice. J Vasc Surg. 2012;55:739–45.

10. Criado E, Johnson G, Burnham S, Buehrer J, Keagy B. Descending thoracic to ilio-femoral artery bypass as an alternative to aortoiliac reconstruction. J Vasc Surg. 1992;15:550–7.

11. Tetteroo E, van der Graaf Y, Bosch J, van Engelen A, Hunink M, Eikelboom B, et al. Randomised comparison of primary stent placement versus primary angioplasty followed by selective stent placement in patients with iliac-artery occlusive disease. Lancet. 1998;351:1153–9.

12. Leville C, Kashyap V, Clair D, Bena J, Lyden S, Greenberg R, et al. Endovascular management of iliac artery occlusions: extending treatment to TransAtlantic Inter-Society Consensus class C and D patients. J Vasc Surg. 2006;43:32–9.

13. Mwipatayi B, Thomas S, Wong J, Temple S, Vijayan V, Jackson M, et al. A comparison of covered vs bare expandable stents for the treatment of aortoiliac occlusive disease. J Vasc Surg. 2011;54:1561–70.

14. Grimme FAB, Goverde PA, Oostayen JA, Zeebregts CJ, Reijnen MMPJ. Covered stents for aortoiliac reconstruction of chronic occlusive lesions. J Cardiovasc Surg. 2012;53:279–89.

15. Fourneau I. How to avoid and manage complications in aorto-iliac interventions. J Cardiovasc Surg (Torino). 2012;53(3):325–31.

16. Jongkind V, Akkersdijk G, Yeung K, Wisselink W. A systematic review of endovascular treatment of extensive aortoiliac occlusive disease. J Vasc Surg. 2010;52:1376–83.

Chapter 4
Upper Limb Ischemia

Lina M. Vargas, Javier A. Alvarez-Tostado, and Daniel G. Clair

Upper Limb Ischemia (ULI)

Upper limb ischemia (ULI) is relatively infrequent when compared to lower limb and accounts for less than 5 % of all extremity ischemia. ULI can be related to a broad spectrum of different etiologies that might require specific therapeutic interventions. Regardless of the etiology, a high index of suspicion and low threshold to initiate treatment are essential for limb salvage.

L.M. Vargas, M.D. (✉)
Department of Thoracic and Cardiovascular Surgery,
Heart and Vascular Institute, Cleveland Clinic,
9500 Euclid Avenue, JJ40, Cleveland, OH 44195, USA
e-mail: linama.vargas@gmail.com

J.A. Alvarez-Tostado, M.D.
Department of Vascular Surgery, Cleveland Clinic,
Marymount Medical Building, Mail Code MT25,
12000 McCracken Road, Suite 351, Garfield, Heights,
OH 44125, USA
e-mail: alvarej3@ccf.org

D.G. Clair, M.D.
Department of Vascular Surgery, The Cleveland Clinic Foundation,
9500 Euclid Avenue, Desk H-32, Cleveland, OH 44195, USA
e-mail: claird@ccf.org

S.K. Shah and D.G. Clair (eds.), *Cleveland Clinic Manual of Vascular Surgery*, DOI 10.1007/978-1-4939-1631-3_4,
© Springer Science+Business Media New York 2014

Large arteries proximal to the wrist are rarely affected while small distal vessels are involved in the majority of cases, comprising around 90 % of all ULI.

Etiology

ULI is caused by diverse entities (Table 4.1) that ultimately lead to vasospasm, obstruction, or a combination of both.

Raynaud's Syndrome

Raynaud's Syndrome is a vasospastic disorder that exhibits an exaggerated response to cold or emotional stimuli (Fig. 4.1). This response induces hand pain, numbness, and color changes from paleness to cyanosis to rubor. It occurs more frequently in upper than lower extremities and is more prevalent in colder climates (15–20 % versus 2–3 %).

1. *Primary Raynaud's Disease*: Abnormal vasospatic response without underlying systemic conditions
2. *Secondary Raynaud's Phenomenon*: Usually associated with an underlying arterial disease or connective tissue disorder with a fixed vascular obstruction and superimposed vasospasm.

TABLE 4.1.   ULI etiologies.

Upper limb ischemia etiologies
1.   Atherosclerosis
2.   Autoimmune/connective tissue disorders
3.   Buerger's Disease
4.   Embolization
5.   Vibration/occupational
6.   Dialysis access steal
7.   Thoracic Outlet Syndrome (TOS)
8.   Trauma
9.   Frostbite

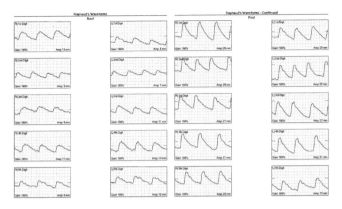

FIG. 4.1.   Reversible vasoconstriction with thermal maneuvers consistent with Raynaud's phenomenon in the left hand.

Connective Tissue Disorders (Scleroderma, CREST, Systemic Lupus Erythematosus)

Usually affects small vessels and is due to cellular proliferation and fibrin deposition that leads to luminal narrowing. Patients can present with symptoms that range from simple Raynaud's phenomenon to frank digit gangrene. In patients undergoing angiography, extensive small artery occlusion affecting arteries of the palmar arch and digits is usually observed.

Occlusive Disease

Occlusive disease is the most common etiology, but only represents <5 % of all cases of limb ischemia.

Atherosclerosis

Usually affects large arteries and arch vessels and frequently is asymptomatic. Diabetic patients and those with chronic renal failure may have an accelerated atherosclerotic process.

Embolic Disease

Embolism is the most common cause of acute upper extremity ischemia and has a cardiac origin in 75 % of patients. The etiology of cardiac emboli is atrial fibrillation in 50 % of cases.

Buerger's Disease

Buerger's Disease is a non-atherosclerotic inflammatory vasculopathy that affects medium-sized vessels primarily (infrabrachial). It is most common in young male smokers, although this pattern is changing as more women smoke. The etiology and pathophysiology remains unclear but is thought to be secondary to an immune reaction that leads to endarteritis and ultimately, thrombotic occlusion of upper- and lower-extremity arteries. In the acute phase, there is neutrophilic inflammation with preservation of the internal elastic lamina, and in the late stage there is perivascular fibrosis and organization of the occlusive thrombus.

Inflammatory Arteriopathies

Takayasu's and Giant Cell Arteritis are the two entities that most commonly affect the upper extremities. *Takayasu's* is the most common and tends to affect the aorta and major branches. Young Asian females are typically affected. *Giant Cell Arteritis* most commonly affects the carotid branches (subclavian and axillary are involved in 10–15 %). Prevalence is higher in older Caucasian females in their 40s and produces visual impairment in 50 % of patients.

Occupational Injuries

These lesions represent cumulative trauma disorders of small vessels. *Vibration-induced White Finger* is the result of repeated trauma-induced vasospasm followed by thrombosis and occlusion of small vessels.

Hypothenar Hammer Syndrome

Repetitive use of palms for pushing, pounding, or twisting that ultimately leads to spasm and/or aneurysmal degeneration of the ulnar artery with microembolization or occlusion. The ulnar artery is most vulnerable at the level of the hypothenar eminence. Occlusive or embolic symptoms are present on the medial aspect of the hand and fingers.

Trauma

Iatrogenic injury of upper extremity arteries can occur during percutaneous access for diagnostic or intervention procedures as well as during catheterization for invasive monitoring. Injuries include hematoma, pseudoaneurysm, occlusion and, or distal embolization. Civilian trauma can be blunt or penetrating.

Arterial Complications of Thoracic Outlet Syndrome (TOS)

Arterial TOS accounts for 1–2 % of all TOS and is the least common when compared to the neurogenic and venous forms. It is due to extrinsic arterial compression that leads to stenosis and post-stenotic dilatation or aneurysmal degeneration. Ultimately, patients can present with embolic events originated from the aneurysm.

Clinical Presentation and Diagnostic Evaluation

Given the multiple etiologic possibilities in a patient presenting with upper extremity ischemia, a detailed and comprehensive history and physical is an essential part of the diagnostic workup. The onset may be acute versus chronic and the duration of symptoms variable depending on the underlying entity. Similarly, signs and symptoms of systemic illness must be noted as they may reveal a patient with risk factors for atherosclerosis, coagulopathy and/or connective tissue disorders such as scleroderma, lupus, or rheumatoid arthritis. Any history of trauma, environmental or occupational exposure must be sought for as patients may not discuss it if they do not think is related to their current complaints.

Physical Exam

Physical examination of a patient with upper limb ischemia should be comprehensive and document pulses in both extremities as well as motor and sensory function. Temperature as well as presence of pallor and other abnormalities such as blue discoloration, ulceration, splinter hemorrhages, telangiectasia, and sclerodactyly must be thoroughly documented. A thorough physical exam should be completed in search for an affected contralateral extremity and other signs of systemic illness, trauma, or exposure.

Laboratory Studies

Laboratory studies are useful in the diagnosis of collagen and connective tissue disorders as well as hypercoagulable states and should be obtained when these entities are suspected.

Noninvasive Testing

1. *Electrocardiogram* may identify abnormal heart rhythms such as atrial fibrillation associated with arterial embolization.
2. *Chest X-ray* may reveal presence of cervical ribs or other bone abnormalities.
3. *Echocardiography* is useful to identify cardiac sources of thrombus especially in patients with rhythm abnormalities or history of myocardial infarction with ventricular wall aneurysms and hypokinesis.

4. *Plethysmography of arms and fingers with segmental pressures* can reveal the level of disease or obstruction as well as any changes after temperature challenges and positional changes such as with TOS maneuvers.

5. *Arterial duplex* is useful to determine the level of disease and determine if there is complete obstruction versus stenosis as well as the presence of possible extrinsic compression such as hematomas.

6. *Computed Tomography Angiography (CTA) and Magnetic Resonance Angiography (MRA)* allows visualization of arterial and venous vessels and determines normal or abnormal anatomy. They are more useful for large arteries proximal to the wrist and preoperative planning.

7. *Angiography* is a useful adjunct to noninvasive testing to confirm a definitive diagnosis. It provides optimal anatomic detail for preoperative planning. Contrast angiography is also useful in patients with small-vessel disease and normal CT angiographic results. Angiography provides information that static studies do not, such as direction of flow, assessment of reconstituted segments, response to vasodilators, and in selected cases has therapeutic potential. Its principal disadvantage is that it is invasive and associated with increased risks when compared to noninvasive testing.

Specific Considerations

Raynaud's Syndrome

1. *Primary Raynaud's Disease*: Usually affects young females more than males and must be present for more than 2 years prior to making the diagnosis.

2. *Secondary Raynaud's Phenomenon* can affect patients at any age and can be seen in both males and females. Unilateral involvement of an extremity is common. Diagnosis is completed with investigation of the arterial system with noninvasive testing or contrast angiography.

Connective Tissue Disorders (Scleroderma, CREST, SLE)

In patients undergoing angiography, extensive small artery occlusion affecting arteries of the palmar arch and digits is usually observed.

Occlusive Disease

Occlusion of palmar and digital arteries is more common than large-vessel disease, and when present, proximal occlusions are better tolerated due to presence of collaterals.

Atherosclerosis

Claudication is the most common complaint when symptomatic, and hand ulceration and tissue loss are rare. Patients may have incidental findings of decreased upper extremity pulses, a blood pressure differential between extremities, and symptoms of vertebral flow reversal due to steal.

Embolic Disease

The site of embolization is the brachial artery in the majority of cases (55 %) followed by axillary (25 %), subclavian (18 %) and forearm arteries (2 %).

Buerger's Disease

Symptoms include pain, claudication, trophic changes, ischemic ulcerations, and gangrene. Other manifestations include Raynaud's phenomenon and superficial thrombophlebitis as it can affect veins too.

Diagnostic workup includes noninvasive testing, and when necessary, angiography can reveal normal proximal arteries with distal occlusive lesions interspersed with normal segments and corkscrew collaterals. There are multiple diagnostic scoring systems such as Shionoya Criteria [1] and Mills & Porter (Oregon) Criteria [2] with slight variations, but the common and most important factors are a history of smoking and exclusion of all other atherosclerotic risk factors except smoking.

Inflammatory Arteriopathies

- *Takayasu's* typically affects young Asian females. Signs and symptoms include headache, fever, joint pain, Raynaud's phenomenon (8–14 %) and ischemic symptoms such as claudication and decreased pulses in the majority of patients (60 %).
- Prevalence of *Giant Cell Arteritis* is higher in older Caucasian females in their 40s and produces visual impairment in 50 % of patients
- Diagnostic workup includes laboratory testing including erythrocyte sedimentation rate (ESR) and noninvasive testing. When pursued, angiography reveals long segments of smooth stenoses with or without post-stenotic dilatation and aneurysmal degeneration.

Occupational Injuries

Vibration-induced White Finger is manifested by blanching and numbness of hands after use of vibrating mechanical tools such as pneumatic hammers and drills. These attacks are short-lived and usually last about an hour and then lead to reactive hyperemia and pain.

Hypothenar Hammer Syndrome

Diagnosis is made on the basis of history and physical examination including the Allen test. Arterial duplex may reveal occlusion or aneurysmal degeneration and contrast angiography is useful for treatment planning.

Trauma

Diagnosis is usually made during physical examination, but depending on the severity and possible associated injuries, a brief bedside evaluation with continuous wave Doppler and Duplex ultrasonography may allow more accurate imaging of the extremity arteries and identify levels of injury. Angiography has a role in certain situations, especially if multiple sites of potential injury are possible, but in general is unnecessary for the diagnosis of vascular trauma. In the majority of cases, the actual injury is determined at time of surgical exploration. Delayed recognition of traumatic arterial injury can lead to pseudoaneurysm or arteriovenous fistula formation.

Arterial Complications of Thoracic Outlet Syndrome (TOS)

Signs and symptoms of arterial TOS include arm claudication, hand ischemia, and Raynaud's syndrome. Noninvasive testing by Duplex, PVRs and segmental pressure measurement with and without TOS maneuvers can aid in the diagnosis.

Management

Management is primarily determined by the underlying etiologic entity.

Raynaud's Syndrome

1. *Primary Raynaud's Disease*: Treatment is based on reassurance and symptomatic control with avoidance of cold temperatures and any identified stressors as well as long-acting vasodilators (nifedipine, losartan).
2. *Secondary Raynaud's Phenomenon*: The treatment encompasses management of any anatomic abnormalities as well as reassurance and education to avoid exposure to cold and stress.

Connective Tissue Disorders (Scleroderma, CREST, SLE)

Treatment includes vasodilators or calcium-channel blockers and adjunctive use of antiplatelet agents. Cilostazol may be beneficial to heal ischemic digital ulcerations.

Occlusive Disease

Treatment options include percutaneous versus open revascularization using vein conduits in the majority of patients.

Atherosclerosis

Since the majority of patients are asymptomatic, most can be followed without interventions and risk factor control with aspirin, statin, and beta-blockers. Interventions include percutaneous angioplasty with or without stenting as well as bypass, usually of proximal vessels like subclavian and axillary arteries.

Embolic Disease

Treatment of acute embolic disease is open embolectomy with anticoagulation unless this is contraindicated. After embolectomy, 95 % of patients will remain free of symptoms. Without anticoagulation one-third of patients will have recurrence. Percutaneous mechanical thrombectomy and thrombolysis are alternatives with comparable success rates to open embolectomy for acute occlusion of large arteries, but with inferior results when small distal vessels are affected. Open embolectomy has been associated with mortality rates as high as 10 % and when the surgical risk is prohibitive, conservative management is associated with significant disability and poor functional outcomes.

Buerger's Disease

Treatment is based on smoking cessation, as no other interventions will be successful if the patient continues to smoke. Supportive treatment with counseling, exercise, wound care, and avoidance of cold temperatures and trauma are essential. Revascularization is a limited option as there are no distal beds for bypass and patency rates are directly linked to smoking cessation. Multiple other interventions such as regional sympathetic block for symptomatic relief, spinal cord stimulation, arterial flow pumps, and even subintimal angioplasty for limb salvage have been tried but all have been fraught with suboptimal results. Appropriate wound care is of utmost importance, and amputation is ultimately required in a number of patients.

Inflammatory Arteriopathies

The basis of treatment is steroid and immunosuppressant medications until symptoms improve and the ESR normalizes. Percutaneous interventions including balloon angioplasty can be attempted but are associated with high rates of restenosis. Surgical revascularization should be delayed until the acute phase is resolved in order to achieve better outcomes and patency rates.

Occupational Injuries

Prevention and removal from the occupation source are essential in the management as well as supportive treatment with reassurance and reinforcement. Revascularization may be attempted in certain patients.

Hypothenar Hammer Syndrome

Avoidance of manual labor and repetitive trauma to the hypothenar region is essential, as well as avoidance of cold temperatures. Vasodilators and calcium-channel blockers may be helpful in some patients. If symptoms persist or are significant, aneurysm resection with or without interposition grafting may be done, and this will ultimately remove the source for microemboli to palm and digital arteries.

Trauma

- *Management strategies* for iatrogenic injuries include open thrombectomy for occlusion and embolization, direct repair versus interposition bypass and evacuation of hematoma. Anticoagulation with intravenous unfractioned heparin might be required in certain situations if not contraindicated by the clinical condition of the patient.
- In cases of injury related to arterial line placement, removal of the line and observation are usually enough as the hand will remain viable due to presence of collaterals, and repair is rarely needed.
- In civilian trauma significant bleeding can occur and is best controlled by direct compression of the injured vessel while allowing collateral circulation to the distal extremity. Tourniquets should be avoided if possible as their use is associated with irreversible upper extremity ischemia and increased rates of amputation.
- Management of blunt or penetrating vascular injuries depends on the extent and location, but the mainstay is to restore perfusion as fast as possible to limit the time of ischemia. Primary repair can be attempted but bypass might be required in certain situations. If the injured segment is short, the vessel can be mobilized and the spatulated ends re-anastomosed. If longer segments are injured, vein or prosthetic grafts can be used. Finally, depending on the location and presence of collaterals, it is possible to ligate an injured artery such as radial or ulnar if the patient has a complete palmar arch (may be incomplete in up to 20 % of patients).
- In cases of multiple musculoskeletal injuries, *arterial repair should occur first* and followed by bone fixation and repair of nerves and tendons. In cases of displacement that might

affect an arterial repair, antegrade perfusion can be achieved by temporary methods such as shunts prior to bone fixation, and definitive arterial repair completed immediately following repair of bone injuries.

Arterial Complications of Thoracic Outlet Syndrome (TOS)

Management of arterial TOS includes first the removal of the arterial compression by resection of the first or cervical rib and division of the anterior scale muscle, second the removal of the source of thrombus by repair of arterial stenosis and resection of aneurysmal segments, and last the restoration of distal circulation by thrombolysis or open embolectomy and in certain situations, arterial bypass.

References

1. Shionoya S. Diagnostic criteria of Buerger's disease. Int J Cardiol. 1998;66 Suppl 1:S243–5.
2. Mills JL, Taylor Jr LM, Porter JM. Buerger's disease in the modern era. Am J Surg. 1987;154(1):123–9.

Chapter 5
Mesenteric Ischemia

Samir K. Shah and Daniel G. Clair

Acute Mesenteric Ischemia

Acute mesenteric ischemia (AMI), defined as hypoperfusion to the intestines, remains a highly lethal disease. Although unified by similar clinical presentation, AMI is caused by diverse etiologies that require specific treatment. Early intervention is critical and physicians must maintain a high index of suspicion.

Clinical Presentation

AMI is heralded by acute-onset continuous poorly localized abdominal pain. Associated gastrointestinal complaints such as diarrhea (42 %), emesis (71 %), and nausea are common.

S.K. Shah, M.D. (✉)
Department of General Surgery, The Cleveland Clinic Foundation,
9500 Euclid Avenue, Desk A100, Cleveland, OH 44195, USA
e-mail: skshah@partners.org; samirkshah.0@gmail.com

D.G. Clair, M.D.
Department of Vascular Surgery, The Cleveland Clinic Foundation,
9500 Euclid Avenue, Desk H-32, Cleveland, OH 44195, USA
e-mail: claird@ccf.org

S.K. Shah and D.G. Clair (eds.), *Cleveland Clinic Manual of Vascular Surgery*, DOI 10.1007/978-1-4939-1631-3_5, © Springer Science+Business Media New York 2014

Pathophysiology

- *Arterial Embolism* to the superior mesenteric artery (SMA) accounts for over 50 % of all cases of AMI. The majority of emboli are cardiogenic, although embolism from more proximal plaque or thrombus has been reported after, for instance, endovascular intervention. It is critical therefore to elicit a history of cardiac disease, especially arrhythmias, infarction, valvular disease, and prior embolic phenomenon. Emboli tend to lodge in distal branches of the SMA leading to sparing of the proximal small bowel and the ascending colon.
- *Arterial Thrombosis* causes 25 % of cases, and typically occurs in the setting of preexisting mesenteric atherosclerotic disease, although only 20 % of patients have had symptoms consistent with prior chronic mesenteric ischemia. Thrombosis tends to occur at the arterial ostium in contrast to embolism.
- *Nonocclusive Ischemia* (NOMI) involves 20–30 % of AMI cases. Central to NOMI is SMA spasm, itself a result of excessive sympathetic outflow. Further, spasm may exist even after treatment of the precipitating event, and reperfusion injury contributes to the final clinical presentation. NOMI is associated with shock, hypovolemia, use of vasopressor agents and digitalis, and cardiopulmonary bypass.
- *Venous Thrombosis* is an often benign condition and accounts for only 1–10 % of AMI. The superior mesenteric and splenic veins are most frequently involved, although it is possible for the portal and inferior mesenteric veins to be affected. Mesenteric venous thrombosis occurs most frequently in patients with hypercoagulable states and prior splenectomy. Onset of abdominal pain may be insidious. As such, a history of these features should increase the index of suspicion.

Diagnosis

- *Physical Exam* is variable. The initial exam may be conspicuous for its lack of findings, leading to the classic early finding of "pain out of proportion to exam," which is absent in 25 % of patients. With ongoing ischemia, the patient may develop ileus and attendant abdominal distention. Transmural infarction with perforation leads to peritonitis.
- *Laboratory* findings are both insensitive and nonspecific. Patients may exhibit leukocytosis, hemoconcentration, elevated transaminases, and amylase. Intestinal fatty acid binding protein is under investigation.
- *Imaging*

  - Plain film—Early cases may demonstrate ileus while late findings include bowel wall edema "thumbprinting" and pneumatosis; 25 % of patients have normal plain films.
  - Duplex ultrasound is not useful in AMI—Although able to visualize SMA and celiac stenoses, its utility is diminished by the presence of intestinal gas in the typical nonfasted patient, and the inability to examine distal branches of the SMA, which are often affected by emboli.
  - Computerized tomographic angiography (CTA)— Multiphase thin-slice CTA has become the default first-line noninvasive imaging modality for AMI with a sensitivity and specificity of 93.3 % and 95.9 %, respectively. It allows adequate visualization of the arterial and venous mesenteric vasculature while allowing assessment of bowel wall edema and enhancement, and alternative etiologies of abdominal pain.
  - Magnetic resonance angiography (MRA)—MRA is not used currently because of poor resolution, inadequate visualization of distal celiac and SMA branches, and overestimation of degree of stenosis.
  - Angiography represents the gold-standard imaging technique and is the only method that allows for simultaneous intervention.

Management

Basic critical care support is the foundation of management and consists of aggressive fluid resuscitation for ongoing third-spacing, broad-spectrum antibiotics to guard against transloca-tion of enteric flora, and heparinization to twice the normal partial thromboplastin time if acceptable. Patients with perito-nitis should receive laparotomy to evaluate for bowel viability and perforation, although cases of laparoscopic evaluation have been described. Otherwise, it is reasonable to proceed first with endovascular evaluation and treatment.

Arterial Embolism

1. *Open Surgery*. Arterial embolism is typically treated with SMA embolectomy. The abdomen is entered via a conven-tional midline laparotomy or bilateral subcostal incision with a midline extension if needed. The bowel is examined first and if there is frank ischemia or perforation, then pro-ceed with resection and control of contamination; other-wise proceed to embolectomy. The omentum and transverse colon are retracted superiorly and the small bowel is retracted inferiorly. The SMA is exposed via an incision made directly over the SMA at the root of the small bowel mesentery. The SMA and its branches are controlled. The SMA is then opened transversely and a proximal embolec-tomy is completed with a 3–4 French (Fr) balloon catheter. There should be pulsatile flow after removal of the embolus. Finally, a distal embolectomy is performed with a 2–3 Fr catheter, taking care to avoid arterial rupture.
2. *Endovascular*. Access may be established via the femoral or brachial arteries. The latter may limit sheath and cathe-ter sizes but facilitates access when the aortomesenteric angle is acute. Initial imaging is completed with a 5 Fr catheter placed at the level of T12. Each visceral artery is then selectively cannulated to identify the target. Contrast is injected and adequate time allowed for filling of small vessels and venous return. The patient is then heparinized and maintained at an ACT of 250–300.

Aspiration thromboembolectomy is then completed. An 8–9 Fr guiding catheter is placed immediately proximal to the embolus, after which a 4–6 Fr guiding catheter is introduced into the embolus. The clot is aspirated with a syringe simultaneous with sheath withdrawal. Several passes are made. Alternatively, specially designed aspiration catheters may be used.

Thrombolysis should be used if there is residual clot or distal emboli. This cannot be used if laparotomy is contemplated and is relatively contraindicated in the presence of bowel necrosis, given the risk of gastrointestinal bleed. The aspiration catheter is left in place and a multisidehole catheter is introduced. Recombinant tissue plasminogen activator 0.5–1 mg/h is infused. Standard lytic care is performed.

Primary stenting with balloon-expandable stents (7–9 mm) is routine.

Arterial Thrombosis

Arterial thrombosis often requires aortomesenteric bypass; simple thrombectomy may be inadequate given coexistent atherosclerotic disease. Prosthetic material is the default conduit, but in cases of contamination or questionable bowel viability, autologous vein is recommended.

1. *Open Surgery*
   Antegrade supraceliac aortomesenteric bypass reduces the risk of conduit kinking and avoids clamping of the infrarenal aorta, which is itself often affected by atherosclerotic disease. The left triangular ligament is divided to allow retraction of the left lateral hepatic segment. The gastrohepatic ligament is divided; after retraction of the esophagus and stomach, the posterior peritoneum is incised to expose the aorta. The celiac and supraceliac aorta are exposed by dissection superiorly. The patient is heparinized (100 u/kg, target ACT 250–300). Side-biting clamps are used to isolate a segment of aorta, in which a vertical aortotomy is made and subsequently used for an end-to-side proximal anastomosis. This is then tunneled behind the pancreas.

The distal anastomosis is made in end-to-side fashion to the distal SMA. Native tissue overlying the aorta and SMA is reapproximated. Risks include worsening of bowel ischemia via supraceliac clamping and compression of the bypass in the retropancreatic tunnel.

Retrograde aortomesenteric bypass provides easier exposure but risks graft kinking and may require iliac or aortic endarterectomy. To expose the SMA, the fourth portion of the duodenum is mobilized. The retroperitoneum overlying the infrarenal aorta and right common iliac artery is exposed. A lazy C bypass configuration is used and the proximal anastomosis is made end-to-end and the distal anastomosis to the iliac artery or distal aorta is made in end-to-side fashion; alternatively, a short graft may be used between the SMA and the infrarenal aorta. Native tissue overlying the aorta and SMA is reapproximated.

2. *Endovascular.* See earlier section on endovascular management of arterial embolism.

Nonocclusive Ischemia

1. *Open Surgery.* NOMI is not treated via open procedures.
2. *Endovascular.* Intraarterial papaverine 60 mg is administered followed by a 30–60 mg/h infusion. Repeat angiography should be performed after 24 h to reassess for NOMI, indicated by narrowing of the origins of multiple branches of the SMA, alternating dilation and narrowing of intestinal vessels along with spasm of the mesenteric arcades, and poor filling of the intramural branches. The infusion may be continued for up to 5 days with ongoing daily angiograms. In case of sudden hypotension, papaverine should be substituted with saline and the catheter position should be confirmed.

Venous Thrombosis

1. *Systemic anticoagulation*, most commonly with unfractionated heparin to a target PTT twice normal, is the first-line treatment where possible to prevent propagation of the

thrombus and may be successful alone in up to 90 % of cases.

2. *Open Surgery* may be contemplated in cases where the patient will be undergoing laparotomy to determine bowel viability. Branches of the superior mesenteric vein may be located at the root of the small bowel mesentery (see previous section on open surgery management of arterial embolism), which may then be traced back to locate it to the right of the SMA at the inferior pancreatic margin. A thrombectomy may be completed with a combination of a Fogarty catheter and milking of the thrombus.

3. *Endovascular.* In cases where systemic anticoagulation appears inadequate and it is necessary to acutely reduce the thrombus burden, aspiration thrombectomy (see earlier section on endovascular management of arterial embolism), chemical thrombolysis (see earlier section on endovascular management of arterial embolism), or device-based mechanical thrombolysis may be used via a transjugular or percutaneous transhepatic approach.

Bowel Viability

Determination of bowel viability, though it may be supported by adjuvant techniques, is ultimately a clinical decision based upon a combination of assessments:

- Clinical indicators of viable bowel include peristalsis, normal bowel color, bleeding from cut surfaces, and palpable pulses along the mesenteric border.
- Fluoroscein injection depends on enhancement of the bowel under ultraviolet exposure to indicate viability. Qualitative interpretation may be difficult.
- Doppler ultrasound of the antimesenteric border.
- A second-look laparotomy should be used to reassess bowel segment in cases of uncertainty to avoid excessive resection and the risk of short-gut syndrome.

Complications

AMI therapy carries significant mortality and morbidity, related to bowel complications and to emergent intervention in high-risk patients (e.g., myocardial infarct, respiratory failure).

- Distal embolization — Small emboli may be clinically inconsequential. Larger emboli should be treated with aspiration embolectomy or thrombolysis
- Vessel dissection — Treat with self-expanding stent placement.
- Access site complications — hematoma and pseudoaneurysm.

Follow-Up

Clopidogrel 150 mg should be given immediately after endo-vascular therapy and then 75 mg daily for 1 month followed by aspirin 325 mg daily for 1 month. Mesenteric duplex ultrasound should be obtained postoperatively to establish a baseline and again at 6 and 12 months thereafter, and ultimately annually.

Chronic Mesenteric Ischemia (CMI)

Clinical Presentation

Most patients are female and will present with dull midepigastric pain occurring approximately 30 min after eating and lasting up to 6 h. Typical patients will have had weight loss of 10–15 kg. Patients may give a history of either constipation or diarrhea. Diagnosis may be complicated by biliary dyskinesia and gastric ulcers, which may be caused by visceral arterial stenosis. Most have a prominent smoking history.

Pathophysiology

Chronic mesenteric ischemia typically results from visceral arterial stenosis resulting in relative postprandial hypoperfusion of the bowel. Normal intestinal circulation receives

10–20 % of the resting cardiac output, increasing to 30 % after eating. Flow-limiting lesions in the vasculature lead to elaboration of ischemic mediators and abdominal pain. Normally, an extensive set of collaterals allows development of symptoms only with disease in two visceral vessels including the SMA; however, destruction of collaterals (e.g., via prior gastrointestinal surgery) may allow symptomatic single-vessel disease. Disease is overwhelmingly atherosclerotic, but may be related to fibromuscular disease, vasculitis, radiation, and drug-effect (e.g., cocaine).

Diagnosis

- *Physical Exam* is nonspecific and generally unhelpful. It is important to note that the absence of findings of systemic vascular disease does not exclude the possibility of CMI.
- *Imaging*:
  - Duplex ultrasound is an excellent tool with two sets of criteria (below). Principal disadvantages are operator dependence and limitations from bowel gas and body habitus.

    Oregon. Peak systolic velocities >200 and 275 cm/s in the celiac and SMA indicates >70 % stenosis. Sensitivity 87–92 % and specificity 80–96 %.

    Dartmouth. End systolic velocity >55 and 45 cm/s in the celiac and SMA indicates >50 % stenosis. Sensitivity 90–93 % and specificity 91–100 %.

  - Computerized tomographic angiography (CTA). Multiphase thin-slice CTA has a sensitivity and specificity >95 % for visceral arterial stenosis. It allows the exclusion of alternative pathologies but at the cost of a higher contrast load relative to angiography. It should be used in patients for whom duplex ultrasound is unavailable and the likelihood of CMI is low.
  - Magnetic resonance angiography (MRA) requires extensive image processing prior to interpretation and

overestimates stenoses. It is not used widely at our institution. Functional studies (e.g., postprandial change in SMV oxygen content and flow), though promising, are not commonly used. 3-D reconstruction sensitivity 100 % and specificity 95 %.

- Endoscopy remains largely experimental.
- Angiography represents the gold-standard imaging technique and is the only method that allows for simultaneous intervention. Disease is most heavily concentrated at the arterial ostia; significant involvement of the distal vasculature suggests a nonatherosclerotic etiology.

Management

Bypass operations offer more durable clinical success (92 % clinical success at 5 years versus 56 % at 2 years [1]) at the cost of higher mortality (13 % at 30 days versus 3.7 % [2]) and morbidity relative to endovascular intervention. Firstline treatment is controversial, but it is reasonable to offer bypass first to younger, appropriate-risk patients.

- *Nutrition*. Patients may be severely nutritionally depleted; such patients should be evaluated for preoperative total parenteral nutrition.
- *Indications* for intervention include symptomatic disease, asymptomatic three-vessel disease, and prior to aortic reconstruction.
- *Target Vessels*. The optimal number of vessels to be revascularized is unclear. Often the SMA alone is treated. In cases of celiac and significant SMA disease (e.g., long occlusion), the celiac should also be revascularized, given the possibility of recurrent SMA disease. The inferior mesenteric artery is not commonly revascularized.
- Open Surgery consists of antegrade or retrograde aorto-superior mesenteric bypass (see earlier section on management of acute mesenteric ischemia), endarterectomy, and arterial reimplantation. Bypass is most common. Prosthetic and autogenous conduits provide comparable results as do antegrade and retrograde bypass.

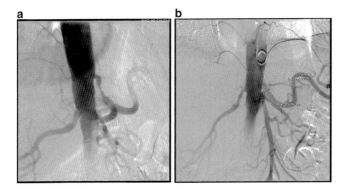

Fɪɢ. 5.1. Angiography for suspected chronic mesenteric ischemia demonstrates (**a**) proximal celiac stenosis and total SMA occlusion, which was treated with (**b**) balloon-expandable stent placement to both vessels with clinical improvement in symptoms.

- *Endovascular*. Access may be established via the femoral or brachial arteries. The latter may limit sheath and catheter sizes but facilitates access when the aortomesenteric angle is acute. Initial imaging is completed with a 5 Fr catheter placed at the level of T12. Selective visceral artery imaging is typically unnecessary. Contrast is injected and adequate time allowed for filling of small vessels. The patient is then heparinized and maintained at an ACT of 250–300. A 6 Fr sheath is advanced to the orifice of the target vessel, and the stenotic lesion is then crossed with an angled hydrophilic wire and 5 Fr angled catheter. The angled catheter should be advanced and position checked. *Primary stenting* with balloon-expandable stents (7–9 mm) of the ostia is routine at our institution (Fig. 5.1). More distal disease should be treated with self-expanding stents.

Complications

- Distal embolization. Small emboli may be clinically inconsequential. Larger emboli may precipitate AMI, and should be treated with aspiration embolectomy or thrombolysis.

- Vessel dissection. Treat with self-expanding stent placement.
- Access site complications. Hematoma and pseudoaneurysm.

Follow-Up

Clopidogrel 75 mg daily for 1 month followed by aspirin 325 mg daily for 1 month. Mesenteric duplex ultrasound should be obtained postoperatively to establish a baseline again at 6 months, and 12 months thereafter, and ultimately annually.

Median Arcuate Ligament Syndrome (MALS)

Clinical Presentation

Most patients are thin young women who present with symptoms of CMI; alternatively, patients may have exercise-induced abdominal pain.

Pathophysiology

The median arcuate ligament is created by crossing fibers from the right and left diaphragmatic crura. An abnormally low diaphragm or superior origin of the celiac artery leads to compression of the latter and rarely the SMA as well. This is exacerbated during inspiration and improves with expiration, when the aorta undergoes physiologic anteroinferior displacement. Celiac compression causes pain via foregut ischemia or a steal phenomenon, wherein blood is diverted from the SMA circulation, leading to midgut hypoperfusion. Recurrent celiac compression by the MAL or by the associated celiac ganglion may lead to pathologic changes in its histologic structure.

Diagnosis

Median arcuate ligament syndrome (MALS) remains a diagnosis of exclusion. Patients should receive a comprehensive evaluation for alternative etiologies of abdominal pain prior to intervention for MALS. Although angiography is the gold standard, duplex US, CTA, and MRA (especially if including 3-D reconstructions) suffice for diagnosis. Asymmetric stenosis of the proximal celiac artery varying with respiration associated with poststenotic dilation is characteristic. Sonography should demonstrate elevated peak systolic velocities that normalize with inspiration and flow reversal within the hepatic artery.

Management

Simple open or laparoscopic release of the ligament along with removal of ganglionic tissue are inadequate treatment given structural changes in the celiac artery. Additional treatment may include aortic reimplantation, patch angioplasty, aortoceliac bypass, or angioplasty/stenting. Endovascular treatment is controversial. Simple angioplasty tends to have high rates of recurrence; stent use risks stent migration and fracture. We prefer to use laparoscopic release of the ligament; angioplasty and selective Nitinol stenting are reserved for selected cases (e.g., failure to improve after release).

References

1. Fioole B, van de Rest HJ, Meijer JR, van Leersum M, van Koeverden S, Moll FL, et al. Percutaneous transluminal angioplasty and stenting as first-choice treatment in patients with chronic mesenteric ischemia. J Vasc Surg. 2010;51(2):386–91.
2. Schermerhorn ML, Giles KA, Hamdan AD, Wyers MC, Pomposelli FB. J Vasc Surg. 2009;50(2):341–348.e1.

Chapter 6
Renovascular Disease

Lee Kirksey

Epidemiology

Renal artery disease includes a group of disorders affecting renal blood flow. Causes of impaired renal blood flow include atherosclerosis, fibromuscular dysplasia, dissection, and trauma. Atherosclerosis is the most common cause of renal artery stenosis (RAS). RAS may be responsible for poorly controlled hypertension and impaired renal excretory function (azotemia). Population-based studies report a prevalence of approximately 7 % in individuals greater than age 65 [1]. In selected populations suffering from peripheral vascular disease, carotid stenosis, and aortoiliac disease the prevalence of RAS may be as high as 40–50 % [2, 3].

Historical Evolution

In 1937, Goldblatt caused hypertension, azotemia, and renal atrophy in a canine model with iatrogenic unilateral RAS [4]. Nephrectomy soon became the treatment of choice for

L. Kirksey, M.D. (✉)
Department of Vascular Surgery, Cleveland Clinic,
9500 Euclid Avenue, Mail Code H32, Cleveland, OH 44195, USA
e-mail: kirksel@ccf.org

S.K. Shah and D.G. Clair (eds.), *Cleveland Clinic Manual of Vascular Surgery*, DOI 10.1007/978-1-4939-1631-3_6, © Springer Science+Business Media New York 2014 renovascular hypertension until a 1956 review of 575 patients revealed a disappointing cure rate of 25 % [5]. Freeman performed transaortic renal endarterectomy in 1954 [6], but a review of results using this technique documented cure in less than half of patients.

Pathophysiology and Clinical Presentation

RAS may manifest clinically as hypertension or renal insufficiency. In general, hypertension directly caused by RAS is associated with refractory, poorly controlled hypertension. Refractory hypertension is defined as at least three classes of maximally dosed antihypertensives—one of which is a diuretic agent.

The degree of azotemia associated with RAS varies from absent to severe owing to associated comorbidities such as diabetes, which may contribute to impaired renal function.

In the early period following the development of hemodynamically significant RAS, the renin-angiotensin-aldosterone (RAA) system is responsible for the body's physiologic response to RAS. Renin produced by the juxtaglomerular cells converts angiotensinogen to angiotensin I. Angiotensin I is converted to angiotensin II (ATII) by angiotensin converting enzyme (ACE). ATII is a potent local and systemic vasoconstrictor. ATII acts on the adrenal gland to promote aldosterone production. Aldosterone is an important mediator of renal tubular sodium absorption and volume expansion. This compensatory effect on volume expansion explains the unexpected worsening in renal function when a patient with bilateral RAS is started on an ACEI or ARB agent. Over time, RAS-mediated volume expansion contributes less to hypertension; it appears that systemic arterial medial wall hyperplasia remodeling is responsible for maintenance of hypertension.

Goals for Procedural Intervention

Although commonly believed that the sole reason for intervening upon RAS is to improve perfusion and halt or improve renal dysfunction, the goals of intervention deserve special attention. Although improvement of renal function or cessation of decline (and thus avoidance of renal replacement) is a laudable clinical benefit, the global focus should be a collective reduction of cardiovascular events (MI, heart failure, and stroke). Selection of the ideal population that benefits from renal revascularization has, and continues to be, the ongoing clinical challenge.

- In carefully selected populations and high volume centers, hypertensive cure rates have been reported to be above 80 % with open dedicated renal revascularization (dedicated suggesting surgery done for isolated RAS and not in combination with aortoiliac [AOI] or aneurysmal pathology).
- For aneurysmal pathology, many centers report morbidity and mortality approaching that for AOI pathology alone.
- For isolated RAS, endovascular therapy is now the most common approach. Contemporary outcomes suggest that 30 % of patients have renal function/hypertensive improvement, 30 % remain the same, and 30 % decline. Postprocedural decline in renal function following catheter-based intervention is attributed to unidentified atheroembolization. It is anticipated that the use of distal embolic protection devices (EPD) may reduce this risk. If EPD is used, one should probably choose a mounted balloon device, which appears beneficial over filters that have pore sizes ranging from 70 to 167 μm.
- Several diagnostic tools help in the selection of ideal candidates and increase the success of renal hypertension intervention. Lateralizing *renal vein renin levels* in the patient with unilateral RAS has an approximately 70 % specificity and sensitivity. A *renal resistive index* (RRI) <0.8 suggests the absence of renal parenchymal fibrotic

changes, an indication of favorable hypertensive response to intervention. The use of these two modalities notwithstanding, *our approach to selecting the patient most likely to benefit* remains based upon clinical features:

- Severe refractory hypertension with optimized and maximized medication dose.
- Pole to pole kidney length >8 cm.
- Progressive and recent decline in renal function.
- Bilateral RAS.
- Flash pulmonary edema.

Open intervention for RAS should be considered in the following cases:

- Children with hypoplastic lesions.
- Concomitant aortic occlusive or aneurysmal disease.
- Branch vessel involvement, i.e., fibromuscular dysplasia (FMD) or multiple small renal arteries not amenable to endovascular intervention.

Imaging

Renal Ultrasound

Renal ultrasound (US) is the imaging *modality of choice*. It is readily available, avoids contrast dye and irradiation, inexpensive, and noninvasive with high specificity and sensitivity when performed in a dedicated, accredited vascular lab. US features of >60 % RAS include:

- Peak Systolic Velocity (PSV) >1.8–2.0 cm/s.
- Poststenotic turbulence.
- Renal aortic ratio >3.5 (ratio of PSVs).
- Pulsus tardus et parvus (decreased and blunted systolic upstroke in the affected artery distal to stenosis).

Computed Tomography Angiography (CTA)

CTA requires contrast in what may be compromised renal function.

Magnetic Resonance Angiography (MRA)

Most MRA protocols require gadolinium, which is contraindicated in patients with chronic kidney disease (CKD) IV/V due to the risk of nephrogenic systemic fibrosis.

Catheter-Based Angiography

Catheter-based angiography permits diagnosis and intervention. Disadvantages include invasiveness and the use of contrast, which can be minimized with the use of carbon dioxide. Complications include access site bleeding and occlusion, and renal parenchymal wire perforation.

Procedural Management

Endovascular

Catheter-based interventions are the most commonly performed approach to isolated RAS occurring in the absence of AOI diseases or aneurysmal aortic disease.

1. The patient should be prepared with intravenous hydration. Randomized trial outcomes are controversial regarding n-acetylcysteine (Mucomyst) and the use of bicarbonate. However, the risks of n-acetylcysteine and bicarbonate are minimal, and we therefore recommend use of these agents. The following agents should be held pre-procedurally: NSAIDs, diuretics, metformin, and warfarin.
2. The site of vascular access is determined based upon preintervention imaging. A femoral approach is frequently used with brachial access reserved for a caudad course of the renal arteries that may be more suitably cannulated from the arm. Benefits of brachial access are weighed against the risk, which is elevated in women and others with small arteries.
3. Diagnostic aortography is performed and pending verification of lesion severity, wire access across the lesion is obtained and the patient systemically heparinized.

(a) Isoosmolar, nonionic contrast is used in dilute volumes to reduce contrast induced nephropathy (CIN). Carbon dioxide angiography is reserved for GFR < 30 ml/min

4. Renal artery occlusive disease is typically spillover from the aorta and represents a bulky aortic plaque origin. Attempts to manage RAS with POBA have been met with a high rate of recoil and lesion recurrence. *Primary stenting* of RAS is now considered accepted practice. For high-grade lesions, predilation with a 3 or 4 mm by 20–30 mm balloon can allow passage of the therapeutic stent. Lesion length typically dictates the use of a 6 or 7 mm balloon expandable stent. The stent is deployed with 1–2 mm protruding into the aorta. After deployment the stent is typically flared to 8 or 9 mm at the renal artery ostium.

Angiography is a two-dimensional modality and thus limited in the context of postdeployment completion evaluation. Alternatives include IVUS to document stent deployment, the absence of residual stenosis, and complete lesion treatment. A residual pressure gradient can be measured with a 4 Fr. catheter pull back over and 0.014 in wire or by using a pressure wire.

Complications

Atheroembolism may occur. Associated factors include:

- Stent oversizing.
- Predilatation.
- Preintervention antiplatelet agent.

Surveillance

Recurrence rates range from 10 to 50 % at 1 year. Postintervention monitoring includes renal US every 4–6 months. Antiplatelet, blood pressure, and cholesterol control is required. Management of recurrent stenosis is dictated by clinical symptoms.

Open Surgery

Options include bypass, endarterectomy, and reimplantation. Of these, bypass and endarterectomy are most commonly performed. In our institution, most operations are performed in combination with aortic intervention. The exposure for intended bilateral RAS includes retraction of the transverse mesocolon cephald and incision of the retroperitoneum. Mobilization of the left renal vein is facilitated by ligation of the iliolumbar, gonadal, or adrenal veins. Wide mobilization of the RA and control with Potts loops are necessary for adequate endarterectomy.

Endarterectomy

If endarterectomy is undertaken, careful completion of an endpoint is the key to success and durable results. Tacking of the endpoint should be performed if there are any questions about plaque stability. After completion and vessel closure, continuous wave handheld Doppler should be used to interrogate the blood vessel assessing for a low resistance, triphasic signal. A water hammer, monophasic signal suggests an untreated flap. Alternatively, high-quality imaging should be sought with vascular lab assistance to conduct the study with the surgeon placing a handheld sterilized probe on the reconstruction and the technician guiding image acquisition.

Bypass

For bypass, an appropriate conduit must be chosen. We favor hypogastric artery for the pediatric patient to reduce the risk of aneurysmal degeneration given durability requirements compared to saphenous vein. For small arteries in the adult, saphenous conduit may be an option. Preoperative assessment and preparing and draping the leg are recommended in any case. The arteriotomy should be 2–2.5 times the conduit size. For most reconstructions, especially when prosthetic is being used for the aortic, 6 mm prosthetic is the conduit of choice. I prefer to perform my graft-renal artery anastomosis first, followed by the aortic anastomosis to facilitate an unfettered, nonkinking path prior to graft transection.

- For isolated ipsilateral RAS treatment on the right, an upper midline, subcostal, or transverse incision allows sufficient access. The falciform ligament is ligated. The right colon is reflected medially after identifying and incising the white line. Ligation of vessels may be required at the hepatocolic ligament. The duodenum is identified and a Kocher maneuver is performed. This allows the head of the pancreas to be reflected medially, revealing the renal hilum, lateral, and medial edge of the IVC.
- The left renal artery may be exposed through the retroperitoneum via a flank or thoracoretroperitoneal incision, a left transverse incision, or an upper midline via the lesser sac.

Renal Fibromuscular Disease

Fibromuscular disease (FMD) is a noninflammatory, nonatherosclerotic disorder that causes arterial wall changes and most commonly affects the renal and carotid arteries. Several variants exist, with the medial being the most common. Less common variants include the adventitial or intimal types.

A typical patient is a woman in her 50s. Most patients are asymptomatic. The pathology is commonly identified incidentally or during an evaluation for other causes of renovascular hypertension.

The lesion has a string or beads appearance on angiography. Grossly web-like intravascular stenosis may alternate with aneurysmal areas. The hemodynamic stenoses cause the associated hypertension. Associated renal artery aneurysms may require treatment based upon size (>3 cm, similar to atherosclerotic renal aneurysms, and those in women of reproductive age).

Treatment is indicated for stenotic, nonaneurysmal lesions in the face of poorly controlled hypertension. Balloon angioplasty without stents has demonstrated better results than those obtained in atherosclerotic renal stenosis. Stents should be avoided. Branch pathology should be considered for bypass given the desire for long-term durability and the fact that the FMD tends to occur in an acceptable medical risk cohort.

Branch vessel open treatment may require ex vivo repair with continuous or intermittent renal perfusion, and syndactylization of the branch vessels on the back table.

Renal Artery Aneurysms

Renal artery aneurysms most commonly are extraparenchymal, saccular, and occur at the main renal artery bifurcation. Patients are typically 40–60 at the time of diagnosis. Hypertension is the most common associated feature, although the relationship is unlikely causal. Repair is recommended at 3 cm in good-risk patients. Anatomy permitting, endovascular therapy may be considered on a case-by-case basis. Open repair through a previously discussed exposure should be considered or ex vivo reconstruction can be done for those that are intraparenchymal.

References

1. Hansen KJ, Edwards MS, Craven TE, Cherr GS, Jackson SA, Appel RG, et al. Prevalence of renovascular disease in the elderly: a population based study. J Vasc Surg. 2002;36:443–51.
2. Missouris CG, Buckenham T, Cappuccio FP, MacGregor GA. Renal artery stenosis: a common and important problem in patients with peripheral vascular disease. Am J Med. 1994;96(1): 10–4.
3. Wachtell K, Ibsen H, Olsen MH, Laybourn C, Christoffersen JK, Nørgaard H, et al. Prevalence of renal artery stenosis in patients with peripheral vascular disease and hypertension. J Hum Hypertens. 1996;10(2):83–5.
4. Goldblatt H. Studies on experimental hypertension: V. The pathogenesis of experimental hypertension due to renal ischemia. Ann Int Med. 1937;11:69.

5. Smith HW. Unilateral nephrectomy in hypertensive disease. J Urol. 1956;76(6):685–701.
6. Freeman NE, Leeds FH, Elliott WG, Roland SI. Thromboendarterectomy for hypertension due to renal artery occlusion. JAMA. 1954;156:1077–9.

Part II
Lymphatic

Chapter 7
Lymphedema

Jeanwan Kang

Introduction

Lymphedema is defined as pooling of protein-rich fluid in the interstitial space due to disruption of lymphatic flow and is classified as primary or secondary, with secondary lymphedema being far more common than primary [1]. Chronic lymphedema can lead to adipose tissue hypertrophy and fibrosis, and rarely lymphangiosarcoma. Treatment consists mainly of nonoperative methods aimed at decreasing edema and preventing recurrent infections.

Anatomy

The lymphatics in the extremities consist of superficial and deep systems, with the former draining the skin and subcutaneous tissue and the latter draining subfascial muscle and bone. In the lower extremities, the two systems merge in the pelvis and drain into the venous system via the thoracic duct. Uptake of interstitial fluid via lymphatic capillaries is

J. Kang, M.D. (✉)
Department of Vascular Surgery, Cleveland Clinic,
9500 Euclid Ave/H32, Cleveland, OH 44195, USA
e-mail: KangJ@ccf.org

S.K. Shah and D.G. Clair (eds.), *Cleveland Clinic Manual of Vascular Surgery*, DOI 10.1007/978-1-4939-1631-3_7,
© Springer Science+Business Media New York 2014

facilitated by local arterial pulsation, skeletal muscle contraction, and unidirectional valves in the lymphatic vessels that prevent backward flow [1, 2].

Classification

Primary Lymphedema is a congenital or inherited condition associated with pathologic development of the lymphatic vessels [3]. Primary lymphedema is classified based on the age of onset as follows:

- *Congenital lymphedema* has onset at birth up to 2 years. Congenital lymphedema is associated with the following conditions:

    - *Hereditary congenital lymphedema* (*Milroy's syndrome*) is an autosomal dominant disease affecting both lower extremities that becomes apparent soon after birth. Lower extremity edema typically does not worsen over time. Most are due to a mutation in the VEGFR-3 gene resulting in impaired lymphatic development.
    - *Cholestasis-lymphedema syndrome* (*Aagenaes syndrome*) is an autosomal recessive disease resulting in congenital lymphatic hypoplasia (decreased diameter of the lymphatic vessels) and recurrent cholestasis.
    - *Other conditions* associated with congenital lymphedema include Noonan syndrome, Turner syndrome, and trisomy 13, 18, and 21.

- *Lymphedema praecox* is the *most common type of primary lymphedema* and has onset between the ages of 2 and 35. It typically presents in girls at the onset of puberty, with unilateral edema mainly involving the foot and calf. There is about a tenfold increase in prevalence in female compared to male. Pathogenesis is unknown in the majority of cases but it is speculated that estrogen may play a role. About 10 % are familial, referred to as *Meige disease*. Meige disease is an autosomal dominant condition and can be associated with double row of eyelashes (distichiasis).

Lymphedema-distichiasis syndrome is due to mutation in the FOXC2 gene (chromosome 16) resulting in agenesis of lymphatic valves and enhanced recruitment of vascular mural cells to lymphatic capillaries. This gene is also highly expressed in venous valves, which may explain why about half of patients with lymphedema-distichiasis syndrome have venous insufficiency.

- *Lymphedema tarda* has onset after age 35. It is more common in women and affects lower extremities.

Secondary Lymphedema is far more common than primary lymphedema and results from acquired lymphatic obstruction or disruption. The most common cause worldwide is filariasis due to infection by the nematode *Wuchereria bancrofti*. In the developed world, cancer (obstruction of lymphatic channels or nodes due to extrinsic compression or tumor cell infiltration of lymphatic vessels, i.e., lymphangitic carcinomatosis) and treatment associated with it (e.g., lymph node dissection, radiation) are the most common causes of lymphedema with breast cancer being the main culprit. Other risk factors for developing secondary lymphedema include older age, obesity, and inflammatory arthritis.

Diagnosis

Diagnosis is based on careful history, physical exam, and exclusion of other causes of limb swelling. About two-thirds of cases of lymphedema are unilateral and therefore patients presenting with bilateral limb swelling should undergo thorough evaluation to exclude other causes of peripheral edema such as chronic venous insufficiency and heart failure. It may be difficult to distinguish between patients with lymphedema from those with chronic venous insufficiency and in some cases the two may coexist. Patients with lymphedema have swelling of dorsum of foot and toes whereas foot swelling is rare in patients with chronic venous insufficiency alone [2]. In addition, lymphedema patients typically do not develop ulcerations [3].

Imaging

Various imaging studies can also aid in diagnosis and include the following:

- Venous insufficiency test to exclude venous insufficiency.
- Computed tomography/magnetic resonance imaging to exclude secondary cause of lymphedema (e.g., tumor).
- Lymphoscintigraphy involves subcutaneous/intradermal injection of radioactive tracers in the web space of the extremities. Imaging is performed 30–60 min following injection. Stress activity (e.g., ambulation, massage) is then performed, followed by repeat imaging. Delayed, asymmetric, or absent visualization of the regional lymph nodes and dermal backflow indicate an abnormal study.

Complications of Chronic Lymphedema

Lymphedema patients are prone to *cellulitis*, which can in turn damage remaining lymphatics. Therefore, timely diagnosis and treatment are imperative in preventing worsening lymphedema. Cellulitis often involves *Staphylococcus* and beta-hemolytic *Streptococcus* infections and the antibiotic of choice is penicillin.

Lymphangiosarcoma is a rare complication of chronic lymphedema. Lymphangiosarcoma following mastectomy is referred to as *Stewart-Treves syndrome*. In patients with lymphangiosarcoma, tumor originates in vascular endothelial cells of the affected limb rather than the lymphatic vessels.

Treatment

Treatment of lymphedema is primarily nonoperative, with the main goal of minimizing swelling and preventing recurrent infections [2–4].

Nonoperative treatment of lymphedema includes a combination of the following:

- Leg elevation.
- Compression stockings (require more compression than in patients with chronic venous insufficiency).
- Pneumatic compression.
- Lymphatic massage, called manual lymphatic drainage.
- Antibiotics for cellulitis.
- Ancillary Medications. Benzopyrones, including coumarin and bioflavonoids, have been shown to reduce lymphedema in some but not all studies.

Surgery is reserved for select patients and should be performed in specialized centers. There are no reasonable-size randomized trials to assess the long-term benefit following these procedures. Surgery can be largely categorized into reconstructive and excisional [5]:

- *Reconstructive* surgery is offered to patients with early-stage lymphedema prior to adipose tissue hypertrophy and fibrosis. They involve lymphatic bypass (lymphatic-lymphatic or lymphovenous bypass), lymph node transfer (microanastomosis of artery and veins with development of neo-lymphatic drainage), and flap transposition procedures (e.g., mobilization of omental flap). Venous hypertension is contraindication to these procedures.
- *Excisional* procedures are offered to patients with advanced lymphedema and are essentially debulking procedures with no improvement in lymphatic drainage. *Charles procedure* involves total excision of all lymphedematous tissues to the fascial level with subsequent skin coverage. The procedure has many wound healing complications and has very limited role in the modern management of lymphedema. Currently, debulking procedures are rarely performed and involve staged excisions with primary closures.

References

1. Warren AG, Brorson H, Borud LJ, Slavin SA. Lymphedema: a comprehensive review. Ann Plast Surg. 2007;59:464–72.
2. Kerchner K, Fleischer A, Yosipovitch G. Lower extremity lymphedema update: pathophysiology, diagnosis, and treatment guidelines. J Am Acad Dermatol. 2008;59:324–31.
3. Lee BB, Andrade M, Antignani PL, et al. Diagnosis and treatment of primary lymphedema. Consensus document of the International Union of Phlebology. Int Angiol. 2013;32:541–74.
4. Rockson SG. Current concepts and future directions in the diagnosis and management of lymphatic vascular disease. Vasc Med. 2010;15:223–31.
5. Gloviczki P. Principles of surgical treatment of chronic lymphedema. Int Angiol. 1999;18:42–6.

Part III
Miscellaneous

Chapter 8
Portal Hypertension

Masato Fujiki, Koji Hashimoto, and Charles Miller

Introduction

Portal hypertension is an elevation of pressure in the portal venous system. It is defined as a portal pressure of >12 mmHg (normal 5–10 mmHg) or a pressure gradient across the liver of >5 mmHg. The causes of portal hypertension can be categorized into prehepatic, intrahepatic, and posthepatic in origin. More than 90 % of portal hypertension is intrahepatic, related to liver cirrhosis. The following discussion reviews the clinical presentation and pathophysiology of portal hypertension and provides an overview of diagnostic techniques and disease management, including discussion of Transjugular Intrahepatic Portosystemic Shunt (TIPS), shunt surgery, and liver transplantation.

M. Fujiki, M.D., Ph.D. (✉) • K. Hashimoto, M.D., Ph.D.
C. Miller, M.D.
Department of General Surgery, Transplantation Center,
Cleveland Clinic, 9500 Euclid Ave. A100,
Cleveland, OH 44195, USA
e-mail: fujikim@ccf.org; masafujiki@yahoo.co.jp;
hashimk@ccf.org; millerc8@ccf.org

S.K. Shah and D.G. Clair (eds.), *Cleveland Clinic Manual of Vascular Surgery*, DOI 10.1007/978-1-4939-1631-3_8, © Springer Science+Business Media New York 2014

89

Clinical Presentation

Clinical history of hepatitis, alcohol abuse, blood transfusion, and family history of liver disease are risk factors for chronic liver disease. Confirmatory evidence of chronic liver disease can be found in various clinical presentations including muscle wasting, jaundice, splenomegaly, spider telangiectasias in the chest wall, and caput medusa. Two major clinical presentations of portal hypertension that require intervention are refractory ascites and esophagogastric varices. Variceal bleeding is the most dreaded complication of portal hypertension and can occur when portosystemic pressure gradient is over 12 mmHg. It carries a 30-day mortality of 20 %. Spontaneous bacterial peritonitis and hepatic encephalopathy are other life-threatening consequences requiring prompt medical management.

Pathophysiology

Table 8.1 provides an overview of portal hypertension by category along with associated diseases and key diagnostic tests.

Prehapatic portal hypertension indicates blockage of the portal or mesenteric vein, mainly due to portal vein thrombosis (PVT). Underlying causes of PVT include liver cirrhosis, tumor thrombus, and, rarely, chronic pancreatitis.

Intrahepatic portal hypertension includes liver cirrhosis and hepatic fibrosis. This can result from a wide variety of etiologies including viral and autoimmune hepatitis, alcohol abuse and toxicity, nonalcoholic steato-hepatitis (NASH), biliary tract disease such as primary biliary cirrhosis and sclerosing cholangitis, as well as a score of less common diseases.

Posthepatic portal hypertension indicates outflow blockage from the liver. Budd-Chiari syndrome implies thrombosis or sclerosis of the hepatic veins and/or the inferior vena cava

TABLE 8.1.   Overview of portal hypertension by category.

Category	Disease	Key diagnostic test
Prehepatic	Portal vein thrombosis	CT
	Congenital extrahepatic portal vein obstruction	CT
	Extrinsic compression of portal vein	CT
	Arteriovenous fistula in portal vein system	CT, US
Intrahepatic	Cirrhosis	Clinical Hx, Lab, CT
	Congenital liver fibrosis	Liver biopsy
	Hepatic sarcoidosis	Clinical Hx, CT, Liver biopsy
	Idiopathic portal hypertension	Liver biopsy
Posthepatic	Budd-Chiari syndrome	US, Hepatic venogram, Hypercoagulable work-up.
	Venooclusive disease	US, Hepatic venogram, Liver biopsy

CT computed tomography, *US* ultrasonography, *Hx* history

(IVC). Fifty percent of Budd-Chiari syndrome is associated with an underlying chronic myeloproliferative disorder (e.g., polycythemia vera, essential thrombocythemia) and an accompanying hypercoagulable state. Work-up for the underlying hematologic disease is necessary. Veno-occlusive disease (VOD) is the occlusion of the terminal hepatic venules and hepatic sinusoids associated with hematopoietic cell transplantation and less commonly with liver transplantation, chemotherapeutic agents, and alkaloid toxins.

Diagnosis

Physical Exam

Ascites is the most common physical finding of patients with portal hypertension. Massive ascites occurs most often in uncompensated portal hypertension. As the body attempts to decompress the elevated pressure, there is a natural response of collateral formation. One type of superficial portosystemic shunt, the caput medusa, can sometimes be seen radiating from the umbilicus as a collateral form from the umbilical vein. A physical examination should include a rectal exam to check for hemorrhoids and the presence of frank or occult blood that can be caused from bleeding from varices in the esophagus, stomach, rectum, and less commonly, other areas of the GI tract. Altered mental status, hepatic encephalopathy, can be seen due to the existence of well-developed, large portosystemic shunts. Current status and history of encephalopathy and the need for lactulose or rifaximin must be assessed carefully since encephalopathy can be exacerbated after the surgical or radiological creation of a new shunt. Uncontrolled encephalopathy is a contraindication for these procedures.

Laboratory

Degree of Portal Hypertension

Thrombocytopenia, along with splenomegaly, is correlated with the degree of portal hypertension. This is known as hypersplenism. Anemia is a common finding in these patients due to chronic liver disease or gastrointestinal bleeding.

Scores to Determine Treatment Options

The Child-Pugh score is widely used to quantify hepatic function reserve, predict prognosis, and select the appropriate surgical intervention. Mortality rates following open abdominal surgery have been reported as 10 %, 17–31 %, and 63–82 % respectively for the patients with Child A, B, and C [1–3]. The Model for End-stage Liver Disease (MELD) score, calculated with total bilirubin, PT-INR, and creatinine, was originally developed to predict the prognoses of patients who undergo Transjugular Intrahepatic Portosystemic Shunt (TIPS) surgery. The MELD score is predictive of 3-month mortality of cirrhotic patients and has been used in the liver allocation system for liver transplant candidates in many countries. It has been suggested that patients with a MELD score below 10 may undergo elective surgery and those with a MELD score greater than 15 should not undergo elective surgery [4].

Hypercoagulable Status

Patients with portal vein thrombosis should be evaluated for hypercoagulable status, including, but not limited to, tests for serum level of protein C, protein S, and antithrombin III, as well as genetic tests for factor V Leiden and JAK-2 gene mutations.

Imaging

Endoscopy

The endoscope is a valuable tool for the screening and treatment of bleeding or nonbleeding varices.

Bleeding varices can be treated with injection sclerotherapy or more commonly variceal band ligation. Band ligation is somewhat more difficult to perform, but has lower morbidity than sclerotherapy and has now become the first-line treatment of choice.

Hepatic Doppler Ultrasonography (US)

Hepatic Doppler US can be used for the screening of thrombosis in the portal and hepatic veins. For the diagnosis of Budd-Chiari syndrome, US has a sensitivity and specificity of 85–90 %. Findings on US consistent with Budd-Chiari syndrome are the absence of flow or thrombosis in the hepatic veins, obstruction of the retrohepatic IVC, and a hypertrophic caudate lobe.

Computerized Tomography (CT) and Magnetic Resonance Imaging (MRI) with Contrast

Triphasic CT with iodine contrast is the best modality to visualize the global picture of the portal venous system and to evaluate the extension of portal vein thrombus. MRI with gadolinium contrast is an alternative for patients who have a history of an allergic reaction to iodine. Compared to an angiogram, CT and MRI provide 3-dimensional information of the anatomy of collateral veins related to adjacent organs and are useful for determining the surgical plan. While contrast CT or MRI can visualize detailed anatomy of collateral vessels, they do not provide information regarding flow volume or direction. In order to evaluate actual flow in collateral vessels, a dynamic angiogram is necessary.

Noncontrast Magnetic Resonance Angiogram (MRA) Without Gadolinium

For patients with kidney dysfunction, image modality options are limited. Triphasic CT with iodine contrast can be performed only when kidney dysfunction is mild and after the patient has had appropriate hydration. However, the administration of iodinated contrast risks further deterioration of renal function due to contrast-induced nephropathy. Additionally, gadolinium contrast for MRI is known to cause irreversible nephrogenic systemic fibrosis, the incidence of which has been reported as up to 7 % for the patient with GFR <30 %.

In these circumstances, noncontrast MRA can help assess the extension of thrombus and the anatomy of collaterals without intravenous administration of gadolinium [5]. Noncontrast MRA provides decent quality, although ascites causes some artifact (Fig. 8.1).

Visceral Angiogram with Portography

A dynamic visceral angiogram through the celiac, superior mesenteric, and inferior mesenteric arteries with a late phase

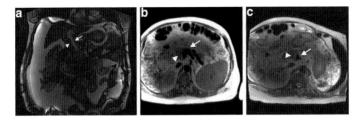

FIG. 8.1. Noncontrast MRA was performed in a patient with kidney dysfunction to assess the extent of portal vein thrombus and the patency of the confluence of splenomesenteric confluence. (**a**) True fast imaging with steady state precession (TrueFISP): Fast flowing blood is *bright* and stationary thrombus is *dark*. *Arrowhead* indicates nonocclusive adherent thrombus. *Arrow* indicates patent portion of main portal and left portal veins. (**b, c**) Single-Shot Fast Spin Echo sequence (HASTE): Fast flowing blood is *dark* and stationary thrombus is *bright*. *Arrowheads* indicate nonocclusive adherent thrombus. *Arrows* show patent splenic and superior mesenteric venous confluence.

portography is performed to assess the flow pattern of the portal vein system. With portal hypertension, main branches of the portal vein system (portal, splenic, gastric, and mesenteric vein) may be separated from each other or connected with little communication due to thrombus or abnormal anatomy. When there are several collateral veins and porto-systemic shunts (e.g., spleno-renal shunt, spleno-retroperitoneal shunt, and gastroesophageal varices), an angiogram with a portogram can show which shunt is the dominant route of collateral flow.

Hepatic Venogram with Pressure Measurement/ Transjugular Liver Biopsy

Wedged hepatic venous pressure (WHVP) reflects the hepatic sinusoidal pressure and therefore the portal pressure. The hepatic venous pressure gradient (HVPG), as measured by hepatic venography, is the pressure gradient between the WHVP and the free hepatic venous pressure, and thus is an estimate of the pressure gradient across the liver.

HVPG measurement is useful to differentiate between prehepatic (normal HVPG), hepatic, and posthepatic causes of portal hypertension (HVPG > 5 mmHg). Additionally, the cavogram with the hepatic venogram is a gold-standard modality to diagnose the Budd-Chiari syndrome and VOD. A hepatic venogram may demonstrate a "spiderweb" pattern diagnostic of Budd-Chiari syndrome. Liver biopsy is nonspecific for Budd-Chiari syndrome, but required for a definite diagnosis of VOD.

Management

Recent advances in the medical and endoscopical management of variceal bleeding have shifted from surgical to non-surgical treatments. However, failure of medical treatment requires interventions such as radiological or surgical shunt creation. These interventions are both palliative and life-saving. Liver or multivisceral transplantation is the ultimate treatment to follow other treatment failures and for patients with Child C cirrhosis [6]. The suggested management algorithm for variceal bleeding is summarized in Fig. 8.2.

Transjugular Intrahepatic Portosystemic Shunt (TIPS)

TIPS is a minimally invasive procedure that provides a direct shunt between the portal and hepatic veins to decompress a high pressured portal system. Because TIPS diverts all portal flow to vena cava, it is considered a nonselective shunt.

Indications

Two well-established indications of TIPS are variceal bleeding that is unresponsive to endoscopical management and ascites that is uncontrolled even when treated with maximized diuretics. In addition, portal hypertensive etiology should be intrahepatic and HVPG should be elevated

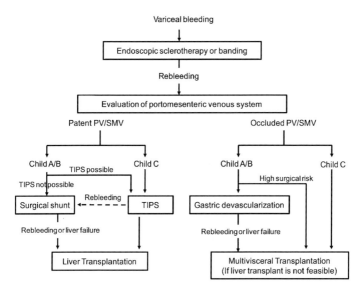

Fig. 8.2. Algorithm for management of bleeding varices. *TIPS* transjugular intrahepatic portosystemic shunt, *PV* portal vein, *SMV* superior mesenteric vein. Algorithm adapted from [6].

(>7–9 mmHg). TIPS is now the preferable choice over a surgical shunt because of the noninvasive nature of the procedure.

A meta-analysis comparison of the efficacy of endoscopic therapy and TIPS in treating acute variceal bleeding showed a significant improvement in hemorrhage control in the TIPS group, but did not show any improvement in overall mortality [7]. With a paucity of data on TIPS, it is recommended to consider this treatment only after medical and endoscopical treatments fail to control acute variceal bleeding.

Patients awaiting liver transplantation frequently have variceal bleeding or refractory ascites and therefore can become candidates for TIPS. Reports show that pretransplant TIPS placement does not affect the outcomes after liver transplantation [8].

Contraindications

Absolute contraindications for TIPS include right heart failure, severe pulmonary hypertension, and polycystic liver disease. Relative contraindications include uncontrolled hepatic encephalopathy, progressive liver failure, and anatomically complicated cases such as large central hepatic tumors, portal vein thrombosis, cavernous transformation of the portal vein, and obstruction of all hepatic veins (advanced Budd-Chiari syndrome) [9].

Recent advances in interventional radiology, however, have made TIPS feasible even for these patients and for those with markedly distorted anatomy such as status post partial liver transplantation with portal vein thrombosis. Before electing TIPS for these high-risk patients, the possibility of rescue transplantation should be discussed. Liver transplantation should be considered when the MELD score is >11 [10] or when cirrhosis-related complications pose a significant risk to the patient.

Complications

The incidence of new or worsening encephalopathy with TIPS is 20–31 %. Rare complications include hemobilia, intraperitoneal bleeding, and hepatic infarction, rating <5 %, 1–2 %, and 1 %, respectively [9].

Follow-Up

Generally Doppler US is recommended to monitor TIPS dysfunction, such as thrombosis and stenosis, although sensitivity of US is unsatisfactory at 10–86 % [11]. An abnormal US finding or recurrent symptoms related to portal hypertension should lead to TIPS venography. Follow-up endoscopy is recommended 1 year after TIPS, especially for the patient with a history of variceal bleeding.

When significant complications occur following TIPS, such as right heart failure, hepatic decompensation, and severe encephalopathy, downsizing or occlusion of TIPS should be considered.

Outcomes

The development of the polytetrafluoroethylene (PTFE)-covered stent for TIPS has significantly improved the stent patency rate at 2 years, up to 76–80 % compared to 19–36 % in bare stents [12, 13].

Despite the improvement in the patency of TIPS, patient survival is suboptimal due to underlying liver disease. The 1-year survival following TIPS for variceal bleeding and for refractory ascites is 48–90 % and 48–76 %, respectively [9].

Shunt Surgery

Surgical shunts can be created between a high-pressure portal vein, or its major branch, and the vena cava, or its major tributary. Surgical shunts are classified as nonselective, selective, and partial, depending on how much portal flow to the liver is preserved.

Nonselective shunts, such as portocaval, mesocaval, and central splenorenal shunts, decompress the total portal system with a wide shunt (>10 mm), thus resulting in a high incidence of encephalopathy. Because of complete diversion of portal flow, accelerated liver failure is the leading cause of mortality following nonselective shunt placement. In an attempt to preserve certain portal flow into the liver and avoid liver decompensation and encephalopathy after the surgery, selective shunts and partial shunts have evolved.

Selective shunts attempt to decompress only the variceal-bearing component of the portal system. The distal splenorenal shunt (DSRS) selectively decompresses the splenic venous system to the left renal vein and disconnects the proximal splenic vein from the portal system [14]. Thus, DSRS preserves high pressure superior mesenteric blood flow to the liver. A small diameter of splenic vein (<7 mm) is not preferable because of a high shunt thrombosis rate.

Partial shunts incompletely decompress the portal system and maintain some hepatic portal flow. Partial shunts can be created with small diameter interposition shunts to 8 mm. A PTFE-reinforced graft is often used as an H-graft between the portal or splenic vein and the vena cava or left renal vein [15].

Indications

Elective shunt surgery is indicated for patients with Child A/B cirrhosis who have recovered from variceal bleeding and are in good condition to undergo a major surgery and are not candidates for TIPS. Emergent shunt surgery is now rarely performed, but still plays an important role in patients who failed endoscopic treatment and TIPS for acute variceal bleeding.

When shunt surgery is required for a future transplant candidate, total portosystemic shunt surgery should be avoided, especially for those who require hepatic hilar dissection. In these cases, surgical difficulty at the time of transplant would be significantly increased.

Contraindications

As mentioned earlier, heart failure, pulmonary hypertension, and uncontrolled encephalopathy are contraindications for shunt creation. Further, shunt creation is not technically feasible for cases of extensive portomesenteric thrombosis. For variceal hemorrhage in patients with extensive mesenteric thrombosis unresponsive to endoscopic treatment, gastric devascularization is an effective, but palliative, treatment and multivisceral transplantation is the only definite treatment [16].

Complications

The incidence of recurrent variceal bleeding and encephalopathy following selective or partial shunt surgeries is reported as 5–8 % and 5–15 %, respectively [14, 17, 18].

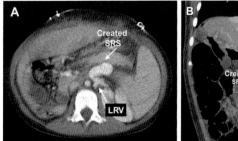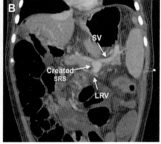

FIG. 8.3. (**a**, **b**) Follow-up CT shows a patent splenorenal shunt (SRS) using H graft between splenic vein (SV) and left renal vein (LRV).

Follow-Up

It is recommended to follow-up shunt patency with appropriate imaging studies prior to discharge from the hospital (Fig. 8.3). Protocol shunt catheterization is not necessary.

Outcomes

Two major clinical trials conducted in the 1990s compared surgical shunts to TIPS using bare stents.

Specifically, a paired randomized trial comparing 66 PTFE 8-mm H-graft portacaval shunt surgeries (HGPCS) and 66 TIPS was initiated in 1993. Half of the study population consisted of Child C patients with a mean MELD score of 14. Study results showed no variceal rebleeding in the HGPCS group compared to 30 % in the TIPS group. Further, the 2-year survival rate was superior in HGPCS group (68 % versus 53 %). Shunt failure was less in the HGPCS group with a re-intervention rate of 11 % versus 48 % in the TIPS group [15].

A randomized multicenter Decompression Intervention of Variceal Rebleeding Trial (DIVERT) comparing 73 DSRS patients and 67 TIPS patients using bare stents was initiated in 1996. The study population consisted of Child A/B patients with a mean MELD score of 9.8. The study showed no significant difference between the two groups in the incidence of rebleeding (6 % versus 11 %), encephalopathy (50 % versus 50 %), and 5-year survival (62 % versus 61 %). However, the reintervention rate was significantly lower in DSRS (11 %) compared with TIPS (82 %) [18, 19].

These studies showed superior patency rates with acceptable survivals in surgical shunts compared to TIPS using bare stents. More recently, covered TIPS stents have gained popularity over bare stents, resulting in a significantly improved patency rate. TIPS is now considered the first-line management and shunt surgery is indicated only in cases where TIPS is impossible or contraindicated.

Liver Transplantation

Liver transplantation is a definite treatment for portal hypertension and is indicated for patients with end-stage liver disease who have failed the aforementioned managements and/or those with Child C or a MELD score greater than 11–15 [10].

Summary

Portal hypertension has various underlying etiologies with the most common being liver cirrhosis, accounting for >90 %. Liver transplantation is the ultimate treatment that addresses both portal hypertension and the underlying liver disease. With the recent advances in the liver transplantation, all liver-related portal hypertensive patients with Child C, MELD > 11, or ascites refractory to medical management should be considered for liver transplantation. Variceal bleeding is the most dreaded complication of portal hypertension and carries a high mortality rate, and thus a prompt management plan is necessary. TIPS is the first choice for recurrent variceal bleeding after endoscopic treatment. Surgical shunts have lost popularity along with the recent advances of interventional radiology and transplantation; however, shunts still play the important role when medical treatment and TIPS both fail to control variceal bleeding.

References

1. Garrison RN, Cryer HM, Howard DA, Polk Jr HC. Clarification of risk factors for abdominal operations in patients with hepatic cirrhosis. Ann Surg. 1984;199(6):648–55.
2. Mansour A, Watson W, Shayani V, Pickleman J. Abdominal operations in patients with cirrhosis: Still a major surgical challenge. Surgery. 1997;122(4):730–5. discussion 735–736.
3. Telem DA, Schiano T, Goldstone R, Han DK, Buch KE, Chin EH, et al. Factors that predict outcome of abdominal operations in patients with advanced cirrhosis. Clin Gastroenterol Hepatol. 2010;8(5):451–7. quiz e458.
4. Hanje AJ, Patel T. Preoperative evaluation of patients with liver disease. Nat Clin Pract Gastroenterol Hepatol. 2007;4(5): 266–76.
5. Lewis WD, Finn JP, Jenkins RL, Carretta M, Longmaid HE, Edelman RR. Use of magnetic resonance angiography in the pretransplant evaluation of portal vein pathology. Transplantation. 1993;56(1):64–8.
6. Costa G, Cruz Jr RJ, Abu-Elmagd KM. Surgical shunt versus tips for treatment of variceal hemorrhage in the current era of liver and multivisceral transplantation. Surg Clin North Am. 2010;90(4):891–905.
7. Luca A, D'Amico G, La Galla R, Midiri M, Morabito A, Pagliaro L. Tips for prevention of recurrent bleeding in patients with cirrhosis: Meta-analysis of randomized clinical trials. Radiology. 1999;212(2):411–21.
8. Bauer J, Johnson S, Durham J, Ludkowski M, Trotter J, Bak T, et al. The role of tips for portal vein patency in liver transplant patients with portal vein thrombosis. Liver Transpl. 2006; 12(10):1544–51.
9. Boyer TD, Haskal ZJ. The role of transjugular intrahepatic portosystemic shunt (tips) in the management of portal hypertension: update 2009. Hepatology. 2009;51(1):306.
10. Englesbe MJ, Schaubel DE, Cai S, Guidinger MK, Merion RM. Portal vein thrombosis and liver transplant survival benefit. Liver Transpl. 2010;16(8):999–1005.
11. Sanyal AJ, Freedman AM, Luketic VA, Purdum 3rd PP, Shiffman ML, DeMeo J, et al. The natural history of portal hypertension after transjugular intrahepatic portosystemic shunts. Gastroenterology. 1997;112(3):889–98.

12. Bureau C, Garcia-Pagan JC, Otal P, Pomier-Layrargues G, Chabbert V, Cortez C, et al. Improved clinical outcome using polytetrafluoroethylene-coated stents for tips: results of a randomized study. Gastroenterology. 2004;126(2):469–75.

13. Bureau C, Pagan JC, Layrargues GP, Metivier S, Bellot P, Perreault P, et al. Patency of stents covered with polytetrafluoroethylene in patients treated by transjugular intrahepatic portosystemic shunts: Long-term results of a randomized multicentre study. Liver Int. 2007;27(6):742–7.

14. Henderson JM, Millikan WJ, Galambos JT, Warren WD. Selective variceal decompression in portal vein thrombosis. Br J Surg. 1984;71(10):745–9.

15. Rosemurgy AS, Bloomston M, Clark WC, Thometz DP, Zervos EE. H-graft portacaval shunts versus tips: Ten-year follow-up of a randomized trial with comparison to predicted survivals. Ann Surg. 2005;241(2):238–46.

16. Abu-Elmagd KM, Costa G, Bond GJ, Soltys K, Sindhi R, Wu T, et al. Five hundred intestinal and multivisceral transplantations at a single center: major advances with new challenges. Ann Surg. 2009;250(4):567–81.

17. Henderson JM, Millikan WJ, Warren WD. The distal splenorenal shunt: an update. World J Surg. 1984;8(5):722–32.

18. Henderson JM. Surgery versus transjugular intrahepatic portal systemic shunt in the treatment of severe variceal bleeding. Clin Liver Dis. 2006;10(3):599–612. ix.

19. Henderson JM, Boyer TD, Kutner MH, Galloway JR, Rikkers LF, Jeffers LJ, et al. Distal splenorenal shunt versus transjugular intrahepatic portal systematic shunt for variceal bleeding: a randomized trial. Gastroenterology. 2006;130(6):1643–51.

Chapter 9
Hemodialysis Access

Lee Kirksey

Chronic Kidney Disease

One in ten American adults, more than ten million people, has chronic kidney disease (CKD) [1]. CKD is defined as a glomerular filtration rate (GFR) of less than 60 ml/min/1.73 m² for more than 3 months or when a patient's urine albumin to creatinine ratio is greater than 30 mg of albumin for each gram of creatinine (30 mg/g).

Epidemiology and Costs

The incidence of patients age 65 and older with CKD more than doubled between 2000 and 2008. End Stage Renal Failure (ESRD) is defined as total and permanent kidney failure. ESRD rates are three times higher for African-Americans compared to non-Hispanic whites. Treating ESRD cost the US more than $40 billion in public and private funds in 2010 [2, 3].

L. Kirksey, M.D. (✉)
Department of Vascular Surgery, Cleveland Clinic,
9500 Euclid Avenue, Mail Code H32, Cleveland, OH 44195, USA
e-mail: kirksel@ccf.org

S.K. Shah and D.G. Clair (eds.), *Cleveland Clinic Manual of Vascular Surgery*, DOI 10.1007/978-1-4939-1631-3_9,
© Springer Science+Business Media New York 2014

Hemodialysis Routes

Routes for hemodialysis vascular access include (1) tunneled dialysis catheter (TDC), (2) prosthetic bridge graft (PBG), and (3) arteriovenous fistula (AVF).

In 1997, the *National Kidney Foundation Disease Outcomes Quality Initiative* (NKF DOQI) [4] set forth a goal of increasing prevalent rates of AVF to 40 % nationally. In 2006, The Fistula First Breakthrough Initiative (FFBI), based upon early progress, modified the prevalent AVF goal to 66 %. Additionally, FFBI set forth a goal of reducing national rates of long-term TDC (i.e., not as a bridge) to less than 10 %. Currently the program's name is modified to *Fistula First/Catheter Last* [5]. In the first year following the initiation of HD, all-cause mortality in ESRD is 20 %. Cardiovascular complications account for 10 % and infectious causes 1–2 %. Extended use of central venous TDC is associated with up to 30 % incidence of significant central vein stenosis. To this extent, early referral with prompt creation of AVF preferably or PBG next can avoid infectious and central vein complications associated with TDC use.

National Trends

Despite broad systemic efforts to identify and refer patients earlier for permanent dialysis access creation, nationally 80 % of patients newly diagnosed with ESRD are initiated on hemodialysis (HD) via a TDC [3]. At 6 months after initiating HD, 55 % of patients continue to be dialyzed with a TDC. Current national rates of AVF are 55 %, PBG 27 %, and TDC 18 %.

Evaluation

History

Obtain information on hand dominance (preferable to use nondominant extremity although vein caliber takes precedence), previous vascular access (central venous catheter, peripherally inserted central catheter, pacemaker, and defibrillator), upper and lower extremity venous thrombosis, hand ischemia, and pulmonary hypertension (potentially exacerbated by arteriovenous fistula).

Physical Exam

- Examine with upper arm tourniquet (note frequently neglected basilic vein).
- Prominent cutaneous chest wall veins.
- Brachial pressure comparison from arm to arm may reveal occult subclavian stenosis. Twenty percent prevalence on left.
- Presence and quality of radial and ulnar pulse. Eighteen to twenty percent overall prevalence of brachial artery variant anatomy. Note also lower extremity pulses.
- Arm circumference. Large circumference may represent a challenge to transposed reconstructions in upper arm and necessitate transposition in the forearm.

Imaging

Noninvasive Vascular Exam

- Duplex venous ultrasound (US) evaluation of the arms and legs, preferably performed by the surgeon. This provides insight into aberrant branching patterns that dictate incision placement. *Vein diameter of 2.5–3.0 mm* is preferred; however the absence of phlebitic or calcific changes is equally important and a 2.5 mm nondiseased vessel is useable.
- Arterial mapping with duplex US evaluation is used to quantify vessel diameter and the absence of calcification. Note the presence of high brachial bifurcations, which is associated with fistula nonmaturation, graft occlusion. The role of corresponding arterial dilation necessary to cause vein maturation is underappreciated and likely explains

the lower rate of maturation in diabetics with fibrocalcific vascular changes.

- Pulse volume recordings (PVR) of the arms or legs in the face of absent pulses, which may be due to noncompressible diabetic calcinosis.

Invasive Testing

I suggest *selective use of venograms* for primary vascular access creation in patients with history of central catheters or stigmata of central venous stenosis given that the rate of stenosis in unmanipulated central veins is low. Whether to intervene prospectively or only if symptoms develop after access creation remains controversial. In patients with preserved renal function CKD IV/V, carbon dioxide with or without a small amount of contrast can allow the central veins to be cleared.

- For secondary access creation in surgical fields that have previously been operated, I routinely perform venography to compliment duplex vein mapping as duplex is less reliable as a standalone modality to evaluate vessel continuity.
- Lower extremity access.

  - There should be a low threshold for arteriography to evaluate diabetics if any physical exam pulse abnormality exists. Otherwise, I insist upon normal PVRs to document normal pedal perfusion.
  - Secondary vascular access evaluation for lower extremity may require CT venography of the iliocaval segment.

Vascular Access Clinical Principles

Contrary to the normal vascular dictum, patency of a vascular access is not the ultimate clinical parameter of success. Anatomic success relies on the *rule of 6s*: 6 mm diameter,

<6 mm below skin, 600 ml/min flow, and 6 cm length of cannulatable vessel. The best conduit is superficial, easily identified, straight, and of large caliber. The ultimate determinant of vascular access success is whether the conduit can be cannulated (14–16 gauge, 3/5–1.0 in. needles). This introduces a level of unpredictability by relying upon the skill of the cannulating technician. Know your center's cannulation team.

Decision-Making Rationale and Options

Based on the overarching theme of Fistula First, start with the most distal autogenous vascular access option.

Radial Artery to Cephalic Vein (Brescia Cimino) Fistula

- High rate of nonmaturation, approaching 50 %, especially in advanced age is likely to be secondary to phlebitic changes due to venipuncture, and so forth.
- May need transposition if it matures but is not able to be seen for cannulation. Veins that will mature should show *30–50 % dilatation at 4 weeks postoperatively*. Consider surveillance vascular access duplex to evaluate for these changes. For absent findings of dilatation, the fistula should be examined carefully for *paraanastomotic flow*, *limiting inflow lesions* (reduced thrill and vein decompresses with elevation of the arm), or *competing accessory veins* (note that the contribution of accessory veins to nonmaturation is not fully agreed upon). In the absence of correctable lesions within the fistula, the vascular access team should have a clear understanding of the threshold to abandon a nonmaturing fistula to proceed to a new site. Poor communication and delayed decision making contributes to avoidable and prolonged use of TDC.

Basic Vein to Ulnar Artery Fistula

Basilic vein to ulnar artery fistula is an oft-neglected option. The vein is frequently preserved and free of venipuncture trauma. However, it must be transposed to the volar surface for patient comfort during dialysis.

Reconstruction

When forearm autogenous access is not available, following FFBI the upper arm should be evaluated for autogenous reconstruction, i.e., cephalic, basilic, or brachial.

- I personally advocate a two-stage approach to upper arm fistula construction with the first stage being primary artery to vein anastomosis through a local incision. Accumulating data are beginning to support the two-stage approach. Several factors explain the higher rate of non-maturation with one stage including warm ischemia to the conduit with dissection from its native vascular bed and blood vessel trauma and subsequent fibrosis in the tunneling/transposition step. I find the conduit produced by the two-stage approach uniformly larger with a much lower rate of nonmaturation and therefore much more easily transposed. Reduced rates of infiltration translate into more durable conduits.

- Because of the prevalence of obesity in our population, it is common to have to transpose a mature cephalic vein as a second-stage procedure, so that it can be identified for easy cannulation. Patients and providers are understanding when informed upfront.

Brachial Artery to Brachial Vein Fistula

For the patient who has limited vein options with regard to the conventional basilic and cephalic approach due to vessel size, I perform a conditioning brachial artery to brachial vein fistula. The brachial vein will either mature along the entire upper arm length and can then be transposed or it will mature at the outflow brachial/axillary vein segment, which will yield a much more durable patency when a bridge graft is constructed at a second stage.

Comparison of Nontransposed Forearm and Upper Arm Fistulas

The present day access literature is evolving to clarify the patency data with new fistula configurations. It is clear that a gold standard for vascular access durability is the Brescia Cimino fistula. After maturation, especially in young patients, this reconstruction may yield a decade of function. The same cannot be expected of transposed reconstructions, which ultimately develop swing point (the anatomic area at upper arm segment of vein where it transitions to the in situ position) lesions likely caused by flow turbulence and mechanical strain. In fact, although much of the literature suggests that the primary patency of the autogenous fistula is significantly better than a bridge graft, the assisted patency benefits are questionable because grafts can be more reliably declotted than fistulas. Transposed vein configurations are durable although they will usually require multiple percutaneous maintenance interventions and should be monitored by an organized surveillance program (i.e., physical exam supplemented with a flow study). That said, the risk of infection with primary fistula (wound infections aside) approaches zero with the subsequent loss of fistula being extremely uncommon. In contrast, the risk of graft infection is 4–5 % and almost always leads to site loss. Clearly the aggregate benefit favors autogenous fistula.

Ipsilateral Axillary Artery-Axillary Vein

When both arms in the infraclavicular location are exhausted, the ipsilateral axillary artery-axillary vein or chest wall "chandelier" represents a novel and neglected option. Because of the high flow arterial and venous flow properties, these constructions are durable. The deleterious impact of this proximal reconstruction on heart disease and pulmonary hypertension should be carefully considered. Requisite is the absence of central venous stenosis. Because "proximalization" is a treatment for steal syndrome, the development of regional hand ischemia is low.

Secondary Vascular Access

Because of the ubiquitous use of TDCs, patients will frequently lose access options due to central vein stenosis/occlusion rendering the upper extremities unusable. Because of this, one should *consider the lower extremities a secondary vascular access option.* The greater saphenous vein because of its usual small caliber (<5 mm) and thicker walls will not dilate and is a poor conduit. The femoral vein with its large caliber is an excellent conduit. It can be mobilized down to the popliteal level and transposed to yield a durable vascular access. A technical pearl is that the vein should be mobilized through an aperture in the sartorius muscle to reduce kinking. Of course, the patient should have normal pedal perfusion and the arteriotomy size should be controlled to limit steal physiology.

- PBG can be performed in the lower extremity if there are limitations for vein use (e.g., DVT, short stature, and limited vein length). The dissection should be carried out at least 5–7 cm below the cutaneous groin crease to limit the rate of infectious complications. In patients with PAD, diabetic vasculopathy, and a predisposition to wounds, the rate of regional steal syndrome is elevated.

Prosthetic Conduit Types

Several options exist for conduit material when nonautogenous reconstruction is created:

- Most common is the use of *expanded polytetrafluoroethylene* (ePTFE). After graft creation, generally 2–3 weeks are required before cannulation can be performed.

This allows incorporation to occur. Incorporation involves the graft becoming densely fibrosed to soft tissues so that when needle cannulation is performed, there is no potential space for hematoma formation.

- A new PTFE-based graft includes the Gore Accuseal™ graft that allows needle cannulation within 24 h by way of a midlayer sealing membrane within a trilayer iteration. I preferentially use this graft in revisions of aneurysmal fistulae that heretofore required a catheter while awaiting incorporation. A similar iteration exists in the Flixene™ graft, which while not FDA approved like the Accuseal™, has been clinically used as an immediate cannulation conduit.
- Bovine carotid artery and cadaveric vein graft have also been used as alternative conduits, although concerns exist about aneurysmal degeneration.

Monitoring

Historically, little has been recommended with regard to surveillance of vascular access despite the improvement in patency that occurs in all other vascular reconstructions that are monitored. My experience is that this too is the case with vascular access. I see patients in follow-up every 3–4 months. I can examine the access for aneurysmal changes, review flow issues, and educate the patient on self-examination. I do not routinely use surveillance duplex for monitoring. The superficial fistula lends itself to examination to reveal pulsatility (outflow stenosis), reduced thrill, or vessel collapse with elevation (inflow stenosis). Monitoring of PBGs is much less reliable and sensitive as the physical exam findings are less appreciable.

Complications

- Infection. <0.5 % with AVF, 4–5 % with PBG.
- Bleeding.
- Venous hypertension. Persistent arm swelling is a sign of central vein stenosis until proven otherwise.

- Ischemic monomelic neuropathy is an uncommon finding of regional complex pain as a result of median nerve ischemia intraoperatively. It is more common in diabetic women with brachial artery-based access and is diagnosed with nerve conduction tests. It should be distinguished from steal and carpal tunnel syndromes.
- Dialysis-associated *steal syndrome* occurs in 1 % AVF and 5–7 % of PBG. This may manifest immediately or after a delay and is more common in women and diabetics, and in those with brachial artery-based access. Diagnosis is inferred by augmentation of radial ulnar pulse or improved Doppler signal with compression of the working fistula or graft and confirmed by a comparison of PVRs with digital pressures with and without access compression.

  - Evaluation consists of angiography from the aortic arch to exclude subclavian artery stenosis and a duplex to evaluate low-flow vs high-flow physiology.
  - Treatment:

    Low flow fistula (<800 ml/min). Proximalization of arterial inflow.

    High flow (>1,000 ml/min). Options include banding, proximalization, revision using distal inflow (RUDI), and distal revascularization with interval ligation (DRIL).

- Congestive heart failure. High-output heart failure is present in 40 % of access patients. It may also be present with a low-flow access when access flow/CO > 0.3
- Pulmonary hypertension. 40–50 % of new-access patients develop new pulmonary hypertension. The arteriotomy size should be limited to prevent the risk of this morbidity, which is also more common with proximal constructions.
- Aneurysm/Pseudoaneurysm.

References

1. Centers for Disease Control and Prevention. 2014 National Chronic Kidney Disease Fact Sheet. http://www.cdc.gov/diabetes/pubs/factsheets/kidney.htm Accessed January 12, 2014.
2. National Kidney and Urologic Diseases Information Clearinghouse (NKUDIC) http://kidney.niddk.nih.gov/kudiseases/pubs/kustats/ Accessed January 12, 2014.
3. U.S. Renal Data System, USRDS 2013 Annual data report: atlas of chronic kidney disease and end-stage renal disease in the United States, National Institutes of Health, National Institute of Diabetes and Digestive and Kidney Diseases, Bethesda, MD, 2013. http://www.usrds.org/adr.aspx Accessed January 12, 2014.
4. National Kidney Foundation Disease Outcomes Quality Initiative (NKF DOQI) http://www.kidney.org/professionals/KDOQI/guidelines_commentaries.cfm Accessed January 12, 2014.
5. Fistula First Breakthrough Initiative (FFBI). http://www.fistulafirst.org/ Accessed January 12, 2014.

Chapter 10
Vasculitis

Carol A. Langford

Vasculitis

Vasculitis is defined by the presence of inflammation within the blood vessel wall. The consequences of vasculitis can include attenuation of the vessel wall resulting in aneurysm formation or vessel rupture or vascular narrowing and occlusion that can lead to tissue/organ ischemia or infarction. Vasculitis is not one single disease and can be seen secondary to an underlying disease or exposure or as a primary vasculitic disease for which the underlying cause has not yet been identified. The vasculitic diseases are rare but potentially organ and life-threatening such that physician suspicion and early diagnosis and intervention are critical.

Vasculitis can occur in blood vessels of any size and one means of categorizing these illnesses has been based upon the predominant size of vessel that is affected [1]. Vascular surgeons may encounter patients with vasculitis who require emergent or elective intervention to address disease involving the medium or large vessels. This chapter will focus on a

C.A. Langford, M.D., M.H.S. (✉)
Department of Rheumatic and Immunologic Diseases,
Center for Vasculitis Care and Research, Cleveland Clinic,
9500 Euclid Avenue A50, Cleveland, OH 44195, USA
e-mail: langfoc@ccf.org

S.K. Shah and D.G. Clair (eds.), *Cleveland Clinic Manual of Vascular Surgery*, DOI 10.1007/978-1-4939-1631-3_10,
© Springer Science+Business Media New York 2014

discussion of the primary vasculitic diseases that are most commonly encountered by vascular surgeons: polyarteritis nodosa, giant cell arteritis, and Takayasu arteritis.

Polyarteritis Nodosa (PAN)

Polyarteritis nodosa (PAN) is defined as a necrotizing arteritis of medium or small arteries without glomerulonephritis or vasculitis in arterioles, capillaries, or venules and not associated with antineutrophil cytoplasmic antibodies (ANCA) [1]. Although PAN was the first vasculitic disease to be described, as it is currently defined it is one of rarest forms of vasculitis with a reported annual incidence rate ranging from 2 to 9 per million. PAN can occur at all ages but is most commonly diagnosed in middle-aged or older adults with a peak in the sixth decade of life. There is a 1.5:1 male predominance. A well-known association exists between hepatitis B and a PAN-like vasculitis. Immunization and the overall reduction in hepatitis B have resulted in a concurrent reduction in occurrence of hepatitis B-associated PAN.

Clinical Presentation

PAN can occur acutely and fulminantly with clinical consequences resulting from vasculitis affecting the medium-sized vessels resulting in stenosis/occlusion with ischemia/infarction or microaneurysm development [2]. The most *common clinical manifestations* of PAN include constitutional symptoms (93 % — fever, weight loss, malaise, night sweats), mononeuritis multiplex (80 %), gastrointestinal (GI) vasculitis (35–65 %), renal involvement (40–50 % — hypertension, renal insufficiency, renal infarction, pericapsular hematoma), skin (50 %), musculoskeletal symptoms (50 %), and involvement of the testicle (15–20 % — pain, infarction), heart (10 % — pericarditis, myocardial infarction, cardiomyopathy), and eye (5–10 %). GI involvement can occur from vasculitis affecting the hepatic, splenic, and mesenteric circulation and represents one of the most life-threatening manifestations [3, 4]. Features of GI involvement can include abdominal pain that can be constant, intermittent, or worse following eating (intestinal angina), bowel infarction and perforation, rectal bleeding, or internal bleeding from microaneurysm rupture. Less common GI manifestations can also include cholecystitis or appendicitis.

Pathophysiology

- *The cause of PAN* remains unknown in the majority of patients.
- *A viral association* in which a PAN-like vasculitis can occur in patients with hepatitis B is readily recognized, but can also occur with hepatitis C, human immunodeficiency virus (HIV), herpes viruses, and parvovirus. In these settings, vessel injury is believed to be related to immune-complex deposition.

Diagnosis

The diagnosis of PAN is made based on compatible clinical features together with evidence supporting vasculitis from either arteriography or vascular histology.

- *Physical Exam* is variable and will be based upon the site of organ involvement. Hypertension can be an important clue to renal involvement. For some organ sites such as the skin, eye, testicle, or nerve, physical examination represents the main means of detecting active disease. A careful abdominal exam is essential in detecting features that might suggest an acute abdomen.
- *Laboratory* findings are nonspecific and there are no laboratory findings that are diagnostic for PAN. Leukocytosis, anemia, thrombocytosis, and elevation of the erythrocyte sedimentation rate (ESR) and/or C reactive protein (CRP) are typically seen consistent with any inflammatory process. Renal findings can include nonglomerular

hematuria, proteinuria, and an elevated serum creatinine. Involvement of the hepatic vessels or an association with hepatitis can result in elevated transaminases. PAN is not associated with ANCA. All patients with PAN should be screened for hepatitis B, hepatitis C, and HIV.

- *Imaging*:
  - *Plain film.* Abnormalities will only be seen in the setting of bowel perforation.
  - *Duplex ultrasound* is not useful in PAN as the vessels involved will be below the level of resolution possible with this procedure.
  - *Computerized tomography* (*CT*) *and CT angiography* (*CTA*). CT can reveal bowel wall edema and alternative etiologies of abdominal pain. CTA is currently not useful in PAN as the vessels involved will be below the level of resolution possible with this procedure.
  - *Magnetic resonance angiography* (*MRA*) is not currently useful in PAN as the vessels involved are below the level of resolution possible with this procedure.
  - *Angiography* represents the *gold-standard* imaging technique for PAN. Characteristic findings include microaneurysms, vessel stenoses, and beading. In patients without contraindications to contrast, mesenteric and renal arteriography should be performed concurrently to increase diagnostic yield as involvement can occur in these locations in the absence of symptoms or signs.

- *Histology*. In some instances, histology from biopsies or surgically removed tissue represents the means of diagnosis. PAN is characterized by *segmental transmural inflammation* of muscular arteries and does not involve veins. The cellular infiltrates consist of polymorphonuclear leukocytes and mononuclear cells. Necrosis of the arterial wall with fibrinoid changes is common. Aneurysmal dilation of the vessel may result from disruption of the internal and external elastic lamina and segmental involvement.

Differential Diagnosis

The differential diagnosis of PAN is broad. Entities to particularly consider include: fibromuscular dysplasia, hypercoagulable states, endocarditis, mycotic aneurysms, atherosclerosis, drug/toxin exposure, segmental arterial mediolysis, and heritable collagen defects such as Ehler-Danlos, Grange syndrome, and neurofibromatosis. Medium vessel vasculitis can also occur in other primary vasculitides and as a secondary vasculitis in connective tissue disease such as rheumatoid arthritis, systemic lupus erythematosus, and Sjögren's syndrome.

Management

Untreated PAN carries a 10 % 5-year survival. Immunosuppressive therapy has dramatically improved outcome increasing the 5-year survival rate to 65–87 % depending on the disease severity. Surgical intervention is only performed in PAN in an acute setting such as where microaneurysm rupture and bleeding have occurred, for an acute abdomen resulting from bowel infarction/perforation or cholecystitis, or in settings such as testicular infarction [3, 4]. As soon as a diagnosis of PAN has been identified, rheumatology consultation should be pursued to assist in medical management.

- Immunosuppression

  - PAN. Determination of the treatment approach in PAN is based upon the degree of disease severity. One instrument used to stratify the severity of vasculitis is the Five Factor Score (FFS). The FFS identifies features associated with a poor prognosis and includes: renal failure (creatinine > 1.58 mg/dL), proteinuria > 1 g/day, cardiomyopathy, central nervous system involvement, and gastrointestinal involvement [5]. Glucocorticoids represent the foundation of treatment in PAN and are used in the spectrum of disease from mild to severe cases. The usual starting dose is prednisone 1 mg/kg/day (not to exceed 60–80 mg/day). This dose is continued for 4 weeks then reduced over the next 6–9 months. Patients who have an FFS=0 can be treated with glucocorticoids alone with close observation for the emergence of severe disease features [6]. For patients with an FFS>1 or with significant mononeuritis multiplex, methylprednisolone 1,000 mg/day for 3 days is often given as the initial glucocorticoid dose followed by prednisone 1 mg/kg/day, which is combined with daily or intermittent cyclophosphamide (CYC) [5]. In studies of severe disease, those treated with CYC were found to have a higher survival rate than those treated with glucocorticoids alone. CYC is typically given for 3–6 months, after which time it is stopped with consideration for use of a maintenance immunosuppressive agent such as azathioprine or methotrexate for the next 1–2 years.

– *Viral associated PAN.* The initial treatment of severe viral associated PAN is similar to that used in PAN but also includes the use of antiviral agents [7]. Once improvement of the vasculitis occurs, immunosuppressive therapy is withdrawn to optimize the ability for antiviral therapy to bring about viral seroconversion. In some studies of hepatitis B-associated PAN, initial use of plasmapheresis was also found to provide benefit.

– *Single organ vasculitis.* There are rare instances of single organ involvement occurring in the gallbladder, appendix, or testicle in which medium vessel vasculitis is found at the time of surgery without evidence of disease elsewhere and for which removal of the affected site is the only required treatment [8]. Such patients should be referred to rheumatology for a thorough evaluation to assure the absence of systemic disease that would require immunosuppression and for ongoing monitoring.

• *Nonmedical intervention.* Although rare, microaneurysm rupture involving the hepatic, splenic, or mesenteric vessels can occur requiring acute intervention. Patients who present with an acute abdomen with features of bowel infarction, bowel perforation, or cholecystitis may also require surgical intervention.

- *Open Surgery.* As microaneurysm rupture is often acute, severe, and life-threatening; an open-surgical approach is usually necessary to control bleeding. Open surgery may also be necessary in the setting of bowel infarction, bowel perforation, cholecystitis, appendicitis, or testicular infarction.
- *Endovascular.* There have been selected reported cases where a bleeding PAN-related microaneurysm has been able to be identified and treated using an endovascular coil embolization [9, 10].

Complications

- *Mortality.* Mortality is influenced by disease severity as seen by a 5-year survival rate of 87 % in those with an FFS = 0 as compared to 65 % in those with FFS ≥ 2 [2]. Most deaths due to active disease occur within the first 18 months. Parameters associated with an increased risk of death include age >65 years, recent onset hypertension, and GI involvement requiring surgery at diagnosis [2].
- *Organ damage.* Despite effective therapeutic intervention, permanent organ damage can still result from irreversible injury that occurred during the initial period of active vasculitis. This particularly includes motor and sensory peripheral nerve damage, renal insufficiency, and hypertension.
- *Treatment-related complications.* Treatment for PAN requires the use of immunosuppression, which itself can be associated with risks of morbidity and mortality. Infection represents the main treatment-related complication and can include bacterial, viral, fungal, and opportunistic organisms. In addition, each agent will have its own specific side effects for which a prevention and monitoring plan must be put into place.

Follow-Up

Patients with PAN require frequent laboratory and physician monitoring to follow the response to treatment, to minimize treatment-related complications, and to watch for evidence of relapse. Relapse has been found to occur in up to 28 % of patients with PAN, which can present in a similar or different manner to the initial presentation.

Giant Cell Arteritis (GCA)

Giant cell arteritis (GCA) is defined as an arteritis, often granulomatous, usually affecting the aorta and/or its major branches, with a predilection for the branches of the carotid and vertebral arteritis with an onset in patients older than 50 years and often associated with polymyalgia rheumatica (PMR) [1]. GCA is the most common vasculitic disease affecting humans, occurring in 26 per 100,000 people. As currently defined, GCA occurs in people over the age of 50 years with an average age in the 70s. There is a 2:1 female predominance with the disease occurring predominantly in Caucasians and persons of European ancestry [11].

Clinical Presentation

GCA is best viewed as a disease possessing four clinical phenotypes: cranial arteritis, PMR, systemic inflammation, and large vessel vasculitis [11]. These features can occur together, sequentially, or distanced by many years.

- Cranial arteritis is the feature most widely recognized with GCA and occurs as the result of vasculitis affecting the internal and external carotid artery and its branches. Symptoms of cranial arteritis include temporal headache, jaw or tongue claudication, scalp tenderness, and visual features. Visual loss is among the most feared complications of GCA and can occur suddenly and may be preceded by transient visual loss or diplopia. Strokes and

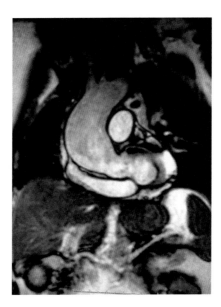

FIG. 10.1. Magnetic resonance imaging demonstrating a 5.0 cm thoracic aortic aneurysm in a patient with long-standing giant cell arteritis.

transient ischemic attacks can be other rare cranial ischemic complications.

- PMR is manifest as aching and stiffness of the shoulder and hip girdles. It can occur in 40–60 % of patients who have other GCA features or in isolation where 10–20 % of patients may at a later time go on to have cranial or large vessel GCA manifestations.
- Features of systemic inflammation commonly accompanies cranial arteritis and PMR and include fever, weight loss, malaise, night sweats, and laboratory features as discussed below.
- Large vessel vasculitis occurs in one-third of patients [12–14]. Long tapered lesions of the subclavian/axillary/brachial arteries are a manifestation affecting one in eight GCA patients. Aneurysms of the thoracic aorta occur in one of five GCA patients and are the most common site of large vessel disease (Fig. 10.1). Thoracic aortic aneurysms

can occur as a late disease manifestation occurring years after the initial disease presentation and are associated with an increased risk of mortality.

Pathophysiology

The *cause of GCA* remains unknown. Evidence from the laboratory supports that GCA is an antigen-driven disease in which macrophages, dendritic cells, and T lymphocytes play a critical role.

Diagnosis

The diagnosis of GCA is made based on compatible clinical features together with evidence supporting vasculitis from either by temporal artery biopsy or large vessel imaging.

- *Physical Exam* is very important in GCA. Head and neck examination should include examination of the scalp and tongue for areas of ischemia and palpation of the temporal arteries for tenderness, nodularity, and pulse. Ocular examination should include assessment of pupillary reactivity and extraocular movements, and any patient with visual symptoms should be referred immediately to ophthalmology for evaluation. A careful vascular examination should be performed to look for signs of large vessel involvement including four extremity blood pressure measurements, examination of peripheral pulses, auscultation for bruits, and abdominal palpation for assessment of the aortic pulse and dimension. Cardiac examination should include auscultation for murmurs. Musculoskeletal examination may reveal tenderness over the deltoid and trochanteric areas and swelling of the peripheral joints can be seen in some patients with PMR.
- *Laboratory* findings are nonspecific and there are no laboratory findings that are diagnostic for GCA. Leukocytosis, anemia, thrombocytosis, and elevation of the ESR and/or CRP are typically seen consistent with any inflammatory process. GCA is not associated with ANCA.

- *Imaging*:
  - *Plain film*. Chest radiograph can provide information about the thoracic aorta. It has been used in some instances as a screening tool to monitor for the development of thoracic aortic aneurysms in patients who have other GCA features but may not be sufficiently sensitive to detect small aneurysms.
  - *Duplex ultrasound* has been used to examine the temporal arteries with description of the "halo sign" as an indicator of vascular inflammation. The utility of temporal artery ultrasound in GCA has been controversial. Although some studies from centers where ultrasound is commonly performed have found this to be useful in guiding biopsy and supporting the diagnosis, other studies have not found this to be any more effective than a thorough physical examination [15, 16]. As the utility of temporal artery ultrasound is heavily influenced by user technique and experience, it is unlikely to have a role in most clinical practices and should not be used as a means of confirming a diagnosis of GCA at this time.
  - *Computerized CT angiography* (*CTA*). CTA can be used to noninvasively visualize the aorta and branch vessels and can provide supportive evidence of large vessel vasculitis. CTA requires contrast and X-ray exposure but remains the preferred technique by some vascular surgeons.
  - *Magnetic resonance angiography* (*MRA*). MRA can also be used to noninvasively visualize the aorta and branch vessels and can provide supportive evidence of large vessel vasculitis. MRA has also recently been used to visualize the temporal arteries. Fat saturated spin echo or gradient echo sequences have been used to examine the vessel wall. While vessel enhancement has been observed in conjunction with edema and inflammation, in Takayasu arteritis this was not uniformly reliable, particularly over serial imaging. At this time, the degree or change in vessel enhancement by MRI should not be used as a measure of disease activity.

- *Angiography* is uncommonly used in GCA due to the availability of noninvasive large vessel imaging techniques via CTA or MRA. Angiography may still have a role, however, when central blood pressure measurements are needed in patients who have four-extremity stenotic disease making peripheral measurements unreliable or for endovascular intervention.
- *Fluorodeoxyglucose positron emission tomography (FDG-PET)*. FDG-PET is a noninvasive imaging technique that visualizes metabolically active tissues. Although primarily used in neoplastic and infection disease settings, large vessel uptake has also been found in GCA. The utility of FDG-PET in GCA remains unclear at this time and is being further investigated.

Histology

Temporal artery biopsy represents the primary means of diagnosing GCA. Biopsy would typically be performed on the symptomatic side, obtaining 2–3 cm of artery. Unfortunately, the positive diagnostic yield of temporal artery biopsies ranges from 50 to 80 % and is even lower in those patients with large vessel presentations. The diagnostic yield may be slightly increased by performing bilateral temporal artery biopsies, but this remains an individual physician decision as to their preference of performing unilateral or bilateral biopsies. In patients where there is a high degree of suspicion for GCA, treatment with glucocorticoids should not be delayed pending the biopsy as histologic changes have been found to persist for weeks after treatment has been started. The histologic findings in GCA include mononuclear cell infiltration involving the adventitia, media, and intima (Fig. 10.2). Multinucleated giant cells, although part of the disease nomenclature, are seen in only 50 % of cases and tend to group around the disrupted elastic lamina.

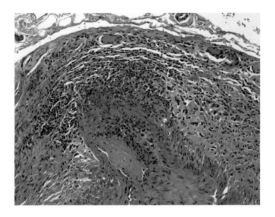

FIG. 10.2. Temporal artery biopsy in a patient with giant cell arteritis demonstrating panmural inflammation.

Differential Diagnosis

The differential diagnosis of GCA is based upon its clinical features. For cranial arteritis this can include thromboembolic disease, other causes of headache, and vision loss. In patients with PMR, the main differential can include rheumatoid arthritis, osteoarthritis, fibromyalgia, and polymyositis. For large vessel disease, this differential would be as described for Takayasu arteritis.

Management

Glucocorticoids represent the foundation of treatment for GCA and are typically combined with low-dose aspirin. Unfortunately, glucocorticoids are associated with a high rate of toxicity and are often required for extended periods of time. To date, no other immunosuppressive agents have been identified as being effective in GCA to treat the disease, reduce glucocorticoid requirements, or prevent relapse. Surgical intervention can play an important role in the setting of large vessel disease.

- *Immunosuppression*
  - *Glucocorticoids.* Since the 1950s, glucocorticoids have been recognized as being effective in reducing not only the symptoms of GCA but more importantly the risk of blindness. Shortly after the introduction of glucocorticoids for the treatment of GCA, the risk of bilateral blindness went from 17 to 9 % and current studies suggest the risk of blindness after starting glucocorticoids to be only 1 % [17]. For this reason, any patient where the diagnosis of GCA is suspected should be started on glucocorticoids immediately to protect vision while the diagnostic evaluation is being pursued. The usual starting dose of prednisone is 40–60 mg/day. This dose is continued for 4 weeks then reduced slowly. There is no widely accepted standard means to reduce prednisone, although one schedule includes a reduction by 5 mg every 1–2 weeks until reaching 20 mg/day then by 2.5 mg every 1–2 weeks until 10 mg/day then by 1 mg every 2–4 weeks. For patients who present with a transient or fixed vision loss, methylprednisolone 1,000 mg/day for 3 days is often given as the initial glucocorticoid dose followed by prednisone 40–60 mg/day. Unfortunately, once vision loss has occurred it is very unlikely to return and the goal of using a methylprednisolone pulse is to protect vision in the remaining eye.
  - *Aspirin.* In two retrospective studies, the use of aspirin was found to be associated with a lower rate of cranial ischemic complications (blindness, stroke) [18]. Although this has not been proven in a prospective trial, the current data supports the use of aspirin 81 mg/day as an adjunctive therapy to prednisone in all patients with GCA who do not have a contraindication.
  - *Other immunosuppressive agents.* Because of the degree of toxicity associated with long-term glucocorticoids, alternative agents have been pursued that reduce the need for glucocorticoids and that reduce relapse. Randomized trials examining methotrexate did not

reduce the rate of glucocorticoid toxicity [19]. Infliximab, a monoclonal antibody directed against tumor necrosis factor (TNF), was found to be no more effective than placebo in reducing relapses and was associated with an increased risk of infection [20]. To date, there remains no therapy beyond glucocorticoids that has been found to be effective in GCA.

- *Isolated aortitis.* There are instances where a patient with a thoracic aortic aneurysm of sufficient size is taken to surgery and unexpectedly found on tissue histology to have evidence of aortitis [21, 22]. In such instances, a careful history should be taken for past or current features of GCA or PMR, acute phase reactants should be measured away from the time of surgery, and vascular imaging by CTA or MRA performed to look for disease in other locations. If there is no evidence by this evaluation to suggest a past or current underlying systemic vasculitis, this would be consistent with a form of single organ vasculitis isolated to the aorta. Such patients with focal idiopathic aortitis may not require glucocorticoids, with the surgical intervention that they have already had being the only required treatment. Such patients should be referred to rheumatology for a thorough evaluation to assure the absence of systemic disease that would require glucocorticoids and for ongoing monitoring.

- *Nonmedical intervention.* Nonmedical interventions in GCA are primarily used to address aortic aneurysms for stenotic lesions causing severe symptoms [23, 24]. Unless intervention is absolutely necessary to protect life or vital organ function, vascular procedures should be avoided when active vasculitis is present and deferred until medical treatment has reduced vessel wall inflammation. The role of perioperative glucocorticoids in clinically quiescent patients remains unclear.

  - *Aortic aneurysm grafting.* In GCA, aortic aneurysm rupture or dissection can occur with smaller size aneurysms if disease activity persists and aneurysms can progress rapidly [23]. The choice of surgical techniques to address aortic aneurysms in GCA does not differ from patients without GCA and depends on the extent of disease. However, involvement of aortic branches in GCA may be more distal, which may increase postoperative complications.

– *Peripheral vascular surgery*. Intervention for upper extremity stenotic lesions should be performed only for extreme claudication affecting quality of life, given the potential for collateral circulation to develop in this location.

– *Endovascular*. Endovascular aortic aneurysm repair (EVAR) can be safely performed in selected patients with GCA [23]. There is less experience with the use of endovascular techniques such as stenting or angioplasty in GCA, but is likely to have low long-term patency rate based on the experience in Takayasu arteritis.

Complications

- *Mortality*. Life expectancy in patients with GCA has been found to remain the same as the general population. Thoracic aortic aneurysms, however, are associated with an increased risk of mortality.

- *Organ damage*. Despite effective therapeutic intervention, permanent organ damage can result from irreversible injury that occurred during the initial period of active vasculitis. Once vision loss has occurred, it is very unlikely to return.

- *Treatment-related complications*. Treatment for GCA requires the use of glucocorticoids, often for extended periods of time. Up to 86 % of patients with GCA have been found to experience one or more glucocorticoid-related adverse events. The older patient population who develop GCA are particularly susceptible to glucocorticoid toxicities that include infections, bone loss, cataract formation, myopathy with increased risk of falls, diabetes, and hypertension.

Follow-Up

Patients with GCA require frequent laboratory and physician monitoring to follow the response to treatment, to minimize treatment-related complications, and to watch for evidence of relapse. Relapse requiring an increase or reinstitution of glucocorticoids occurs in 70–90 % of patients with GCA. While this often presents with PMR, cranial, or inflammatory symptoms, late onset large vessel disease represents a potential relapse manifestation of GCA. In patients with known large vessel disease, vascular imaging by CTA or MRA should be performed every 6–12 months and for the development of new clinical features. For patients who do not have large vessel involvement, the optimal monitoring beyond physical examination remains unclear, although annual chest radiography to monitor the thoracic aortic shadow has been advocated by some investigators.

Takayasu Arteritis (TAK)

Takayasu arteritis (TAK) is defined as an arteritis, often granulomatous, predominantly affecting the aorta and/or its major branches, with a predilection for the branches of the carotid and vertebral arteritis with an onset in patients younger than 50 [1]. TAK is an uncommon disease occurring in three per one million people. As defined, TAK occurs in people younger than the age of 50 years with an average age in the 20s. There is a 9:1 female predominance in patients from Japan and the United States, although nearly equal representation in men and women has been seen in other countries. TAK may have a varying spectrum in different populations but is seen throughout the world.

Clinical Presentation

In 10–20 % of patients with TAK, there are no presenting features and evidence of disease is found incidentally. The remaining 80–90 % of patients present with features of

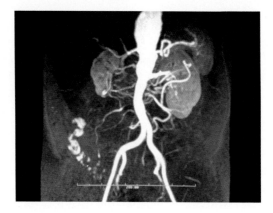

Fɪɢ. 10.3.   Magnetic resonance imaging in a patient with Takayasu arteritis demonstrating an aneurysm of the abdominal aorta with marked reduction in size of the right kidney due to renal artery stenosis.

systemic inflammation (fever, weight loss, malaise, night sweats) and/or vascular symptoms. Vascular symptoms occur as a direct reflection of the location of the stenotic or aneurysmal disease and the tissues being provided by this blood flow [25, 26]. The subclavian artery is usually the most commonly affected vessel during the patient's course (20–78 %) with stenosis resulting in upper extremity claudication. Renal artery involvement (15–50 %) can result in hypertension and renal insufficiency (Fig. 10.3). Involvement of the carotid and vertebral arteries can manifest with central nervous system hypoperfusion symptoms including transient ischemic attack (TIA), stroke, syncope, visual changes, dizziness, and hearing loss. Involvement of mesenteric vessels is common but frequently asymptomatic due to collateral flow. Thoracic aortic aneurysms can result of aortic root dilation and aortic valvular insufficiency.

Pathophysiology

The cause of TAK is unknown.

Diagnosis

The diagnosis of TAK is made based on compatible clinical and large vessel imaging features where other etiologies have been excluded.

- *Physical Exam* in TAK focuses on the vascular examination including four extremity blood pressure measurements, examination of peripheral pulses for presence or tenderness (particularly carotidynia), auscultation for bruits, and abdominal palpation for assessment of the aortic pulse and dimension. Cardiac examination should include auscultation for murmurs. The remainder of the examination continues to be important, particularly following diagnosis in examining for evidence of therapeutic toxicity.
- *Laboratory* findings are nonspecific and there are no laboratory findings that are diagnostic for TAK. Leukocytosis, anemia, thrombocytosis, and elevation of the ESR and/or CRP are typically seen consistent with an inflammatory process. TAK is not associated with ANCA.
- *Imaging*:
    - *Plain film*. Plain films do not have a clear role in TAK.
    - *Duplex ultrasound* has been used as a noninvasive technique to examine peripheral vessels. It has a limited role in TAK at this time.
    - *Computerized CT angiography* (*CTA*). CTA can be used to noninvasively visualize the aorta and branch vessels and can provide supportive evidence of large vessel vasculitis. CTA requires contrast and X-ray exposure but remains the preferred technique by some vascular surgeons.
    - *Magnetic resonance angiography* (*MRA*). MRA can also be used to noninvasively visualize the aorta and branch vessels and can provide supportive evidence of large vessel vasculitis. MRA has also recently been used to visualize the temporal arteries. Fat saturated spin echo or gradient echo sequences have been used to examine the vessel wall. While vessel enhancement has

been observed in conjunction with edema and inflammation, this is not uniformly reliable, particularly over serial imaging [27]. At this time, the degree or change in vessel enhancement by MRI should not be used as a measure of disease activity.

– *Angiography* is uncommonly used in TAK due to the availability of noninvasive large vessel imaging techniques via CTA or MRA. Angiography may still have a role, however, when central blood pressure measurements are needed in patients who have four extremity stenotic disease making peripheral measurements unreliable or for endovascular intervention.

– *Fluorodeoxyglucose positron emission tomography (FDG-PET)*. FDG-PET is a noninvasive imaging technique that visualizes metabolically active tissues. Although primarily used in neoplastic and infection disease settings, large vessel uptake has also been found in GCA. The utility of FDG-PET in TAK remains unclear at this time and is being further investigated.

Histology

Vascular histology is uncommonly used as a means of diagnosis for TAK but may be obtained at the time of vascular procedures. The histologic findings in TAK include panarteritis that typically occurs as focal skip lesions. The inflammatory infiltrate is predominantly lymphocytic with granuloma formation and giant cells involving the media and adventitia. Later, degeneration of the internal elastic lamina of the media, adventitial fibrosis, and neovascularization occur.

Differential Diagnosis

The differential diagnosis of TAK includes: atherosclerosis, IgG4-related disease, fibromuscular dysplasia, infectious aortitis, and heritable collagen defects such as Marfan syndrome, Ehler-Danlos, Loeys-Dietz, neurofibromatosis, and pseudoxanthoma elasticum. Large vessel vasculitis can also occur in other primary vasculitides and as a secondary vasculitis in inflammatory bowel disease, sarcoidosis, and spondyloarthritis.

Management

Glucocorticoids represent the foundation of treatment for TAK. Although other immunosuppressive agents are commonly used in TAK, this is based solely on open-label studies. Surgical intervention plays an important role in TAK to address stenotic or aneurysmal disease causing significant symptoms.

- *Immunosuppression*
  - *Glucocorticoids*. Glucocorticoids have been found to improve systemic symptoms and improve blood flow in some patients [25]. The usual starting dose of prednisone is 1 mg/kg/day (no higher than 60–80 mg/day). This dose is continued for 4 weeks then reduced over the next 6–9 months. For patients who present with severe ischemia due to vessel stenosis or occlusion, methylprednisolone 1,000 mg/day for 3 days is often given as the initial glucocorticoid dose followed by prednisone 60–80 mg/day.
  - *Aspirin*. The data with aspirin in TAK is less than in GCA. In one study of 48 patients, aspirin had a protective effect with a low frequency of bleeding complications [28]. Although this has not been proven in a prospective analysis, the use of aspirin 81 mg/day should be considered in patients with TAK who do not have a contraindication to this.
  - *Other immunosuppressive agents*. Because of the degree of toxicity associated with long-term glucocorticoids, the young age of these patients, and high rate of relapse with TAK, alternative immunosuppressive agents have been pursued. Although other agents are commonly used in TAK, all experience gathered with these has some from open-label studies. To date, there has been

no randomized studies performed that has demonstrated any agent to be more effective than glucocorticoids alone. Methotrexate 15–25 mg/week is commonly used and has been found to be of benefit in open-label studies of relapsing disease [29]. As it is teratogenic, women of child-bearing potential should be screened for pregnancy before this is started and counseled regarding the need for effective contraception. Recent retrospective series has also suggested a benefit with TNF-inhibitors, such as infliximab [30]. Other agents for which there has been open-label experience include mycophenolate mofetil and azathioprine. CYC is rarely used and only for severe life-threatening disease, largely due to the young population that is affected by TAK and the potential for infertility with CYC.

- *Hypertension*. Treatment of hypertension represents among the most important interventions in TAK in reducing renal, cardiac, and cerebral risk. Upper extremity blood pressure measurements may not be representative of aortic root pressure because the subclavian arteries are a frequent site of vessel stenosis. When treating hypertension, care should be taken to avoid rapid drops in blood pressure, particularly in patients with compromised cerebral blood flow.
- *Isolated Aortitis*
See previous section discussing Giant Cell Arteritis management: isolated aortitis.
- *Nonmedical Intervention*
Nonmedical interventions are important in TAK for the revascularization of stenosed or occluded vessels that produce significant ischemia or for the treatment of aneurysms [23, 24, 31, 32]. Up to 70 % of patients with TAK arteritis may require nonmedical interventions, with the most frequent indications including cerebral hypoperfusion, renovascular hypertension, coronary artery disease, severe limb claudication, repair of aneurysms, and valvular insufficiency. Intervention should not be performed on asymptomatic lesions. Intervention for upper extremity lesions should be

performed only for extreme claudication, given the potential for collateral circulation to develop in this location. Unless intervention is absolutely necessary to protect life or vital organ function, vascular procedures should be avoided when active vasculitis present and deferred until medical treatment has reduced vessel wall inflammation. The role of perioperative glucocorticoids in clinically quiescent patients remains unclear.

– *Aortic aneurysm grafting.* The choice of surgical techniques to address aortic aneurysms in TAK does not differ from patients without TAK and depends on the extent of disease [23].

– *Peripheral vascular surgery.* The safety and potential benefits of vascular reconstructive surgery in patients with TAK have been favorable. However, occlusion and complication rates vary widely between series. Current studies suggest that vascular bypass surgery carries a higher rate of patency over time compared with endovascular approaches [31, 33, 34]. The site of revascularization is also important with regard to the long-term outcome, and care should be taken to avoid placing surgical connections to vessels that are frequently known to become involved during the course of disease. Grafts for involved cervicobrachial vessels should ideally originate from the ascending aorta because this segment rarely becomes stenotic.

– *Endovascular.* Endovascular approaches for vascular stenotic lesions with angioplasty or stents have been attractive because of their less invasive nature. The short-term results have been encouraging, but some series have found a high rate of restenosis or occlusion over extended follow-up. A possible exception has been seen with the use of stent grafts for TAK, which appears to be associated with better long-term patency results [35]. Further data will be needed to understand the durability and role of this endovascular therapy in these patients. EVAR has been successfully used in selected patients with TAK.

Complications

- *Mortality*. The outcome of patients with TAK has varied between studies. In two North American series, a 95 % long-term survival was seen, but in other studies the 5-year mortality rate has been as high as 35 %. Disease-related causes of mortality include cerebrovascular events, myocardial infarction, congestive heart failure, aneurysm rupture, or renal failure.
- *Morbidity*. TAK is associated with substantial morbidity and disability. In one series, 74 % of patients exhibited compromised function in activities of daily living and 47 % were permanently disabled.
- *Treatment-related complications*. Treatment for TAK requires the use of immunosuppression, which itself can be associated with risks of morbidity and mortality. Infection represents the main treatment-related complication and can particularly include bacterial, viral, and opportunistic organisms. In addition, each agent will have its own specific side effects for which a prevention and monitoring plan must be put into place. As TAK affects young patients who wish to pursue child-bearing, the potential for teratogenicity needs to be considered.

Follow-Up

Patients with TAK require frequent laboratory and physician monitoring to follow the response to treatment, to minimize treatment-related complications, and to watch for evidence of relapse. Relapse occurs in 70–80 % of patients with TAK. This may be manifested by systemic inflammation or new vascular lesions in new territories. Vascular imaging by CTA or MRA should be performed every 6–12 months and for the development of new clinical features.

References

1. Jennette JC, Falk RJ, Bacon PA, et al. 2012 revised international Chapel Hill consensus conference nomenclature of vasculitides. Arthritis Rheum. 2013;65(1):1–11.
2. Pagnoux C, Seror R, Henegar C, et al. Clinical features and outcomes in 348 patients with polyarteritis nodosa: a systematic retrospective study of patients diagnosed between 1963 and 2005 and entered into the French Vasculitis Study Group Database. Arthritis Rheum. 2010;62(2):616–26.
3. Levine SM, Hellmann DB, Stone JH. Gastrointestinal involvement in polyarteritis nodosa (1986-2000): presentation and outcomes in 24 patients. Am J Med. 2002;112(5):386–91.
4. Pagnoux C, Mahr A, Cohen P, et al. Presentation and outcome of gastrointestinal involvement in systemic necrotizing vasculitides: analysis of 62 patients with polyarteritis nodosa, microscopic polyangiitis, Wegener granulomatosis, Churg-Strauss syndrome, or rheumatoid arthritis-associated vasculitis. Medicine (Baltimore). 2005;84(2):115–28.
5. Gayraud M, Guillevin L, le Toumelin P, et al. Long-term followup of polyarteritis nodosa, microscopic polyangiitis, and Churg-Strauss syndrome: analysis of four prospective trials including 278 patients. Arthritis Rheum. 2001;44(3):666–75.
6. Ribi C, Cohen P, Pagnoux C, et al. Treatment of polyarteritis nodosa and microscopic polyangiitis without poor-prognosis factors: a prospective randomized study of one hundred twenty-four patients. Arthritis Rheum. 2010;62(4):1186–97.
7. Guillevin L, Mahr A, Callard P, et al. Hepatitis B virus-associated polyarteritis nodosa: clinical characteristics, outcome, and impact of treatment in 115 patients. Medicine (Baltimore). 2005;84(5):313–22.
8. Hernández-Rodríguez J, Molloy ES, Hoffman GS. Single-organ vasculitis. Curr Opin Rheumatol. 2008;20(1):40–6.
9. Parent BA, Cho SW, Buck DG, et al. Spontaneous rupture of hepatic artery aneurysm associated with polyarteritis nodosa. Am Surg. 2010;76(12):1416–9.
10. Stambo GW, Guiney MJ, Cannella XF, et al. Coil embolization of multiple hepatic artery aneurysms in a patient with undiagnosed polyarteritis nodosa. J Vasc Surg. 2004;39(5):1122–4.
11. Salvarani C, Pipitone N, Versari A. Clinical features of polymyalgia rheumatica and giant cell arteritis. Nat Rev Rheumatol. 2012;8(9):509–21.

12. Bongartz T, Matteson EL. Large-vessel involvement in giant cell arteritis. Curr Opin Rheumatol. 2006;18(1):10–7.
13. Kermani TA, Warrington KJ, Crowson CS, et al. Large-vessel involvement in giant cell arteritis: a population-based cohort study of the incidence-trends and prognosis. Ann Rheum Dis. 2013;72(12):1989–94.
14. García-Martínez A, Arguis P, Prieto-González S, et al. Prospective long term follow-up of a cohort of patients with giant cell arteritis screened for aortic structural damage (aneurysm or dilatation). Ann Rheum Dis. 2013 Jul 19.
15. Schmidt WA, Kraft HE, Vorpahl K, et al. Color duplex ultrasonography in the diagnosis of temporal arteritis. N Engl J Med. 1997;337(19):1336–42.
16. Salvarani C, Silingardi M, Ghirarduzzi A, et al. Is duplex ultrasonography useful for the diagnosis of giant-cell arteritis? Ann Intern Med. 2002;137(4):232–8.
17. Aiello PD, Trautmann JC, McPhee TJ, et al. Visual prognosis in giant cell arteritis. Ophthalmology. 1993;100(4):550–5.
18. Nesher G, Berkun Y, Mates M, et al. Low-dose aspirin and prevention of cranial ischemic complications in giant cell arteritis. Arthritis Rheum. 2004;50(4):1332–7.
19. Hoffman GS, Cid MC, Hellmann DB, Guillevin L, et al. A multicenter, randomized, double-blind, placebo-controlled trial of adjuvant methotrexate treatment for giant cell arteritis. Arthritis Rheum. 2002;46(5):1309–18.
20. Hoffman GS, Cid MC, Rendt-Zagar KE, et al. Infliximab for maintenance of glucocorticosteroid-induced remission of giant cell arteritis: a randomized trial. Ann Intern Med. 2007; 146(9):621–30.
21. Rojo-Leyva F, Ratliff NB, Cosgrove 3rd DM, et al. Study of 52 patients with idiopathic aortitis from a cohort of 1,204 surgical cases. Arthritis Rheum. 2000;43(4):901–7.
22. Liang KP, Chowdhary VR, Michet CJ, et al. Noninfectious ascending aortitis: a case series of 64 patients. J Rheumatol. 2009;36(10):2290–7.
23. Albacker T, Svensson L. Cardiothoracic surgery for Takayasu's arteritis and ginat cell arteritis. In: Hoffman GS, Weyand CM, Langford CA, Goronzy JJ, editors. Inflammatory diseases of blood vessels. 2nd ed. Oxford: Wiley-Blackwell; 2012.
24. Rajani RR, Kashyap VS. Peripheral vascular surgery for large vessel vasculitis. In: Hoffman GS, Weyand CM, Langford CA, Goronzy JJ, editors. Inflammatory diseases of blood vessels. 2nd ed. Oxford: Wiley-Blackwell; 2012.

25. Kerr GS, Hallahan CW, Giordano J, et al. Takayasu arteritis. Ann Intern Med. 1994;120:919–29.

26. Maksimowicz-McKinnon K, Clark TM, Hoffman GS. Limitations of therapy and a guarded prognosis in an American cohort of Takayasu arteritis patients. Arthritis Rheum. 2007;56:1000–9.

27. Tso E, Flamm SD, White RD, et al. Takayasu arteritis: utility and limitations of magnetic resonance imaging in diagnosis and treatment. Arthritis Rheum. 2002;46(6):1634–42.

28. de Souza AW, Machado NP, Pereira VM, et al. Antiplatelet therapy for the prevention of arterial ischemic events in Takayasu arteritis. Circ J. 2010;74:1236–41.

29. Hoffman GS, Leavitt RY, Kerr GS, et al. Treatment of glucocorticoid-resistant or relapsing Takayasu arteritis with methotrexate. Arthritis Rheum. 1994;37:578–82.

30. Molloy ES, Langford CA, Clark TM, et al. Anti-tumour necrosis factor therapy in patients with refractory Takayasu arteritis: long-term follow-up. Ann Rheum Dis. 2008;67:1567–9.

31. Liang P, Tan-Ong M, Hoffman GS. Takayasu's arteritis: vascular interventions and outcomes. J Rheumatol. 2004;31:102–6.

32. Giordano JM, Leavitt RY, Hoffman GS, et al. Experience with surgical treatment for Takayasu's disease. Surgery. 1991;109:252–8.

33. Kim YW, Kim DI, Park YJ, et al. Surgical bypass vs endovascular treatment for patients with supra-aortic arterial occlusive disease due to Takayasu arteritis. J Vasc Surg. 2012;55:693–700.

34. Saadoun D, Lambert M, Mirault T, et al. Retrospective analysis of surgery versus endovascular intervention in Takayasu arteritis: a multicenter experience. Circulation. 2012;125:813–9.

35. Qureshi MA, Martin Z, Greenberg RK. Endovascular management of patients with Takayasu arteritis: stents versus stent grafts. Semin Vasc Surg. 2011;24:44–52.

Index

S.K. Shah and D.G. Clair (eds.), *Cleveland Clinic Manual
of Vascular Surgery*, DOI 10.1007/978-1-4939-1631-3,
© Springer Science+Business Media New York 2014

Printed by Printforce, the Netherlands